'In this carefully crafted, wide-ranging book, Ruth Phillips demonstrates fully what it means to think, live, and work as a feminist (Mama, 2020). *Practising Feminism for Social Welfare* is a real contribution to the development of feminist theory and practice across the world'.

Viviene E. Cree, *Emerita Professor of Social Work Studies,*
The University of Edinburgh, UK

PRACTISING FEMINISM FOR SOCIAL WELFARE

There has been an explosion of interest in feminism in recent years. This book argues it is still necessary and has a vital role. Feminism's core objectives – to address the persistent issue of women's inequality and ongoing sexism, and to fight against women's oppression and improve women's lives – remain of central value across the world. As a result, how feminism contributes to and improves social welfare is overdue for re-examination.

This text explores what feminism means in theory, policy and practice as it is conceptualised and engaged within different social welfare contexts today. Beginning with an overview of feminist scholarship in the 21st century, it mainly comprises six substantive chapters that examine feminism from within a specific policy or practice setting. The topics discussed include globalisation and social justice, motherhood and reproductive rights, domestic violence, women's experiences in criminal justice settings and working with older people. *Practising Feminism for Social Welfare* concludes with a framework for feminist policy and practice in the era of the fourth wave, whilst acknowledging that there can be no single or hegemonic feminism across all sites of social and political processes and in all social welfare settings.

Designed as an introduction to feminist practice for social policy and social work audiences, this volume will also speak to a range of academic disciplines, including sociology, criminology, politics, women's studies, and gender and feminist studies.

Ruth Phillips is an Associate Professor in Social Work and Policy Studies at the University of Sydney. With a practice background in social policy in government and feminist and environmental activism, Ruth teaches social policy in social work and global social policy as well as having supervised many PhD students, particularly from the South-East and East Asian region. She has published widely in her areas of research, which includes third sector studies, social policy and feminism in social work.

PRACTISING FEMINISM FOR SOCIAL WELFARE

A Global Perspective

Ruth Phillips

Routledge
Taylor & Francis Group

LONDON AND NEW YORK

Cover image: © Getty Images

First published 2023
by Routledge
4 Park Square, Milton Park, Abingdon, Oxon OX14 4RN

and by Routledge
605 Third Avenue, New York, NY 10158

Routledge is an imprint of the Taylor & Francis Group, an informa business

© 2023 Ruth Phillips

British Library Cataloguing-in-Publication Data
A catalogue record for this book is available from the British Library

Library of Congress Cataloging-in-Publication Data
Names: Phillips, Ruth, author.
Title: Practising feminism for social welfare: a global perspective / Ruth Phillips.
Description: 1 Edition. | New York, NY: Routledge, 2023. | Includes bibliographical references and index. |
Identifiers: LCCN 2022030254 (print) | LCCN 2022030255 (ebook) | ISBN 9781138650671 (hardback) | ISBN 9781138650688 (paperback) | ISBN 9781315625188 (ebook)
Subjects: LCSH: Feminism. | Feminist theory.
Classification: LCC HQ1155 .P45 2023 (print) | LCC HQ1155 (ebook) | DDC 305.4209—dc23/eng/20220818
LC record available at https://lccn.loc.gov/2022030254
LC ebook record available at https://lccn.loc.gov/2022030255

ISBN: 978-1-138-65067-1 (hbk)
ISBN: 978-1-138-65068-8 (pbk)
ISBN: 978-1-315-62518-8 (ebk)

DOI: 10.4324/9781315625188

Typeset in Bembo
by codeMantra

Dedicated to my closest feminist allies,
my sons Eugene and Reuben and my partner Michael.

CONTENTS

Preface   *xi*

1   Feminism as Praxis   1

2   Global Feminism, Global Social Policy and Social Welfare   22

3   Domestic Violence: Feminism and Feminist Practice   44

4   Feminist Practice, Motherhood, Trans Parenthood and
    Maternal Rights   71

5   Reproductive Justice, Rights and Welfare, the Role of
    Feminist Practice   100

6   Older and Old Women and Feminist Practice   124

7   Feminist Perspectives on the Criminal Justice System
    and the Law   150

8   Conclusion: The Fourth Wave and Feminist Practice   176

Index   *189*

PREFACE

Ideas for this book have been heavily influenced by the period of writing and have changed and developed along the way. The stepping back of my co-author due to health reasons early in the piece, the death of my mother, the rapidly changing university environment in which I work, which created piles of new demands in how we work, and global political, environmental and social transformations are factors that have, to some extent, dictated the direction of the book. This was especially the case in the period close to finalising the manuscript when the global novel coronavirus pandemic created major disruptions in everyone's lives, both from a personal perspective due to being drawn away from this project in the work context and also more directly as it affected the lives of women and their loved ones around the world. The years 2019, 2020, 2021 and 2022 will forever be marked by the pandemic, and for many people, it will take years to recapture some form of equilibrium in their lives.

It has also been an important time in history when the Black Lives Matter movement gained momentum and brought the lived experiences of deeply entrenched racism into the global public eye. Although sparked in the USA, focusing on systematic police brutality and an increasingly overt white supremist political culture, the wildfire of resistance and outcry resounded around the world. In that response, it was evident that there are still many people who recognise solidarity as a core value for human well-being, and the diverse support for the Black Lives Matter movement showed us that social movements can bring people together for a better world. However, it was also an important reminder to anyone who identifies as a feminist that we (white feminists) too have acted in ways that have not only excluded women of colour, often argued as unthinkingly, but also harmed and oppressed women of colour in our efforts in striving and fighting for our equality and ideas of equality. I cannot and do not seek to speak for women of colour, nor do I seek women of colour to help me in my work. I do, however, defer to the expertise and research of women of colour and First Nations Peoples that has produced insightful knowledges born from diverse struggles and offer alternate ways of viewing the world to my own. Such perspectives reflect differing life experiences of women and of feminists across the world. It is my hope that by including examples of feminists' engagement and action as, and with, social welfare practices that have affected diverse women from diverse contexts, a global perspective of feminist praxis can be illuminated.

So, this is a white feminist's book and I acknowledge that white feminism has been largely a response to white patriarchy. Where women of colour and First Nations People's experiences are included as examples of feminist practice, they will often reflect the impact of white patriarchy either directly through dominant global North economic or social impositions or historically because of colonisation. This is a particularly important position for me as a white Australian, and I acknowledge the critical work of First Nation Australians who have 'spoken up' to white feminists, who have rightly pointed out that the failure to work alongside Indigenous women and women of colour meant we were participants in First Nations women's oppression, therefore part of the white patriarchal colonial oppressions experienced since colonisation. Here I refer particularly to the critical analyses by Aileen Morton-Robinson (2000), Lillian Holt (1993), Christine Fejo-King (2016) and the many other Indigenous women who have faced and fought many deeply entrenched white privilege-driven impositions. It is an important and salutary reflection to recognise that power can be abused within a movement or as part of a theorisation of how to change the world. Many might argue that this was never a conscious act, but white privilege and its racist impact are most often exercised 'unconsciously'. This happens because we are part of the hegemony of dominant social, political and economic assertions of a far-reaching global North and predominantly white culture, a culture that has disallowed other cultures to be recognised as equal and as sources of equally important knowledge. I also acknowledge that the English language is never going to be adequate in representing women across the world and that strategically feminism is not always used to describe feminist practice. As Amina Mama notes in relation to African women:

> It is still an African commonplace to attribute anything concerning women, rights, peace, and development to 'feminism'… in ways that situates it as a dangerous foreign interference, racialized white, and sexualized lesbian. It therefore makes little sense to focus our attention on whether women activists in Africa name themselves 'feminist' or not. From a movement perspective we need to tend to what the term means among the community of women who think, live and work as feminists on the continent and value the work that we do.
>
> *(2020, p. 363)*

What is important about how I have been positioned, as the author, by direct and indirect events is that in a book about feminist praxis, both the personal and the political are always intertwined and bound to the lived experience of practicing and thinking about feminism. I also recognise that despite the times I have had to be resilient, I have always been secured and protected by my white privilege and the economic security of my economic class. To that end I see my role in producing this book as creating a reflective opportunity for readers to consider the intersection of feminism and social welfare as a demonstration of how to apply and exercise a feminist lens. This is based, to some extent, on my own feminist practice but mostly on researching and seeking to understand the very wide forms of feminist practice across the world, not as a scholarly expert but rather as a fellow traveller with other feminist activists, thinkers, researchers, scholars and social welfare practitioners.

References

Holt, L. (1993) One aboriginal woman's identity: Walking in both worlds. *Australian Feminist Studies*, 8 (18), 175–179.

Mama, A. (2020). "We will not be pacified": From freedom fighters to feminists. *The European Journal of Women's Studies*, 27 (4), 362–380.

Morton-Robinson, A. (2000) *Talkin' Up to the White Woman: Aboriginal Women and Feminism*. St Lucia: University of Queensland Press.

Tedmanson, D. and Fejo-King, C. (2016) Talking up and listening well, dismantling whiteness and building reflexivity. In S. Wendt and N. Moulding (eds) *Contemporary Feminisms in Social Work Practice* (1st ed.), 149–165. London: Routledge.

1

FEMINISM AS PRAXIS

Introduction

This chapter introduces key ideas in the book and outlines what is to come in further chapters. I begin by acknowledging that feminism is not a monolithic concept or practice but can be seen as having emerged as several ideologically determined theories and action with a *shared over-arching purpose* and residing in or alongside intellectual commitments and political movements. These multiple forms of feminism have sought social justice and equality for women, thereby calling for an end to sexism in all its forms and, as Shaw puts it, 'the development of consciousness of sexism and the willingness to join with others to end discrimination against women' (2015, p. 167). Feminisms also acknowledge that gender is a key organising principle and see the human world as largely organised by gender and difference and, as I argue throughout and emphasise in the final chapter, have evolved to be more inclusive of diverse sexual identities. I think that feminism, despite its internal battles for meaning and nuance in practice, can be seen as a framework for social justice activism that seeks equality for all oppressed groups. I will use the term throughout the book to describe the collective efforts of all feminists engaged in thought and practice who apply a feminist (however it maybe be defined) lens, regardless of the site or means of that practice. I also believe that feminist identification is not the corollary of feminist practice, you don't have to say 'I am a feminist' to act in a feminist way. After all, feminism emerged historically as a form of resistance to systematic and personal oppressions and exclusions of women, manifested in their inferior status compared to men across most cultures, resulting in an uneven hold on political, social, economic, religious and personal power between genders. This rather elastic idea of feminism, as will be developed further in later chapters, allows for the broad scope of the book, in terms of both feminism and social welfare, and

DOI: 10.4324/9781315625188-1

hopefully opens opportunities for understanding the purpose, goals and impact of feminism on social welfare.

Setting broad parameters does not mean that the complexity of feminist thought will be ignored or denied as one of the most positive aspects of feminism is its continual evolution and contextual responsiveness, provoking and absorbing self-reflexive critique and constant, persistent external backlashes and resistance to how it may change interpersonal relationships, social and economic structures, and politics. Beyond this, feminism is the subject of much debate, theorisation and controversy, both within and outside feminism itself and, most importantly, is a form of articulated and developed practice across the broad terrain of welfare, social policy and everyday life. It is the realisation that feminism is theory-and-practice ('praxis'). Even in the cases where global North feminisms are seen to and do oppress women of colour or global South women, there are synergies in the objectives of local feminists from vastly diverse ethnic, religious and national cultures and that is what I have hoped to capture in this book.

Feminism is something that is 'done' by feminists across the world. It is about understanding the world and then trying to change it – as Liz Stanley wrote more than 32 years ago, 'the point is to change the world, not only to study it' (1990, p. 15). Indeed, feminism, from a very broad perspective, has changed the world, with a lasting impact. This was evident in a report in *The Lancet* about a University of Washington study, which examined the projected changes in population growth and the decline of populations in countries such as China, Japan, Thailand, Spain and others, which are predicted to halve by 2100 (Vollset et al., 2020). Such countries have already been affected by low birth rates, related to reproductive choice and one suggested reason from the authors of the study was:

> "We've realised there's something different about our species, namely that women can control their fertility," he says. "And as they get more educated and have access to jobs and careers they choose to have fewer children than replacement requires."
>
> *(Safi, 2020)*

It also appears that countries where feminist activity has been suppressed and deep patriarchal frameworks continue to affect reproductive choice, through religious and far-right ideologies, will be sites of population growth over the next 80 years (Safi, 2020).

Feminism has been influential because, like patriarchy (men's systematic assertion of power over women and non-binary gendered people, through control of institutions, laws and the economy) or neoliberalism, it is also something that is, quite literally, 'practiced' – it does not stay the same, and it reflects the changing ideas and context within which it is situated. Although often perceived as an action/theory of political and social resistance set up to gain equality in a world dominated by men and masculinity, it also exists within the solidarity of women from the grassroots level of families and matriarchal cultures, in communities, organisations and even institutions such as feminised workplaces, particularly in social welfare. Lombardo and Verloo (2009) wrote about procedural feminism, where they sought to move away from types of feminism to focus on the processes that characterise feminism. They argue that this procedural definition of feminism 'allows not only the hegemonic struggle with various types of gender inequality (or patriarchy) to be taken onto account, but also encompasses hegemonic struggles within feminism' (Lombardo and Verloo, 2009, p. 109). There is a strong similarity between feminism as praxis, as applied throughout this book, and procedural feminism.

The process of collective knowledge building and drawing on lived experiences has been both the practising of resistance and of critique, and as Gunew pointed out, this process gave rise to the tensions 'between the commonality of women's experience and its diversity, based on race, class, religion and age etc.' (1990, p. 24). This inevitably led to diverse groups of women having to resist and challenge the dominance of white middle-class women speaking on their behalf and continues to be a dynamic interaction within feminism. What is important about the tensions within feminism is that they have resulted in shifts in all spheres of feminist practise and theory. For example, the current omnipresent, fourth wave, idea of intersectional feminism (Phillips and Cree, 2014) within activism and research has allowed the structural concerns of radical feminism to be informed by an intersectional view of the lived experience of women, which is inclusive of diverse and often multiple aspects of that experience. But what is often theoretically adjusted does not necessarily result in gains for minority groups as the wider demands for women are often only rarely met in the most general terms and often still fail to be met via social policy, particularly in the context of the dominance of neoliberalism and economic rationalism. In turn, this means that hard fought for gains in services for women will be seen to be failing groups of women who have specific needs for support such as LGBTQI people, women with disabilities or women of colour. Although 'intersectional' feminist theory and practice can be seen as an adjustment in feminism, in recognition of diversity in identity and needs, there is still a more inclusive feminist practice being demanded of dominant middle-class white women who are seen to be benefitting most from their efforts and their privilege. Of course, this not an absolute distinction and there are a range of ways that dominant feminisms and feminist services have been inclusive of diversity or have provided useful tools, strategies, and mechanisms for diverse groups to utilise in their own struggles (Eyadat, 2013; Ramirez, 2007).

It is, however, this omnipresence and the ever-changing and ever-growing quality of feminism that both inspires and intrigues feminist researchers, teachers and activists and is a key motivation for writing this book. Hence this book will not recount in detail the wide theoretical history or roots of feminism as so many scholars have done before. Neither will it seek to explain the highly developed contemporary theorisations of feminism, except when it is necessary to highlight the theory practice nexus to illuminate why some feminists do things differently from other feminists. It is also necessary when feminist debates or theories prompt certain public responses or activism that are motivated by a theoretical impasse or debate. Hence the content of each chapter aims to build knowledge about some key social welfare issues that feminist practices and action must and do encounter today. This knowledge has been gathered from feminist research, feminist commentary, feminist action, feminist activism, reporting on feminism and my experiences of practicing, researching and teaching feminism within the broad landscape of social welfare and social policy. As stated above, a key component of writing as a feminist is recognising that as the author/writer I must constantly reflect on my own positionality – as a tail-end baby boomer, as white, as privileged (with education and a successful working life) and as a mother.

Also, part of my privilege as an academic and an activist for positive social change has meant I have travelled extensively and engaged with social and political issues from a global perspective in my teaching and my research. Therefore, this book is based on a premise of seeing the world from a global perspective and drawing on knowledges and experiences from both the global South and the global North. This perspective of feminism also shares theoretical frameworks with postcolonial analysis that is strongly evident in Indigenous peoples' resistance to colonial, mostly white impositions. This is highly pertinent for social welfare in much of the world and as observed by Tedmanson and Fejo-King (2016, p. 150) a

> shared sense of postcolonial feminist ethics challenges us to extend our concern for women's oppression to a deepening awareness of the multi-layered oppressions experienced by Indigenous women whose knowledges, cultures and languages must be repositioned to the centre of all professional discourse.

The lasting impact of colonisation underpins engagement with global South perspectives and examples of feminist practice in this book in an effort to reposition the place of knowledges from the South against the hegemonic bulwark of global North theory and ideas. Further, since the relatively recent, heightened recognition of the power of globalisation, it is hoped that readers of this book recognise the interconnectedness of social problems and the importance of interconnected networks that fight for social change but also what we can learn from actions, struggles and successful transformations in other geographical, social and cultural places.

In this era, the 2010s and the 2020s, it has been clear in the public sphere that there has been a visible emergence/re-emergence of interest in feminism per se across the global North and global South. This interest is igniting and re-igniting debates around gender equality and women's rights and roles and opening new discussions about the nature of feminism itself and how and who it can serve as a politics for social change. It has also resulted in an increase in the practice of feminism arising in many sites of political and social change, human services and social policy governance across the world. This book will be both an exploration and analysis of some of the many sites where feminism is being practiced across the world. In doing so important, contextual elements such as the role of social media, the dominance of neoliberalism and the rise of state-based economic austerity in the industrialised world, a new generation of young people encountering sexism, the recent rise of populist and nationalistic politics and wider international events such as the global Corona Virus pandemic, which have forced women's status onto the public agenda will form the backdrop. I also engage with the concept of transformations in contemporary feminism as praxis and the potential and possibilities of a fourth wave of feminism, which is the focus of the concluding chapter.

Importantly, feminist debates, observations and research are seen more as a means than an end. Feminism, when practised, is done as part of an over-arching framework for social justice and a key hope of this book is to add to strategies that will achieve greater social justice on a broad scale and more specifically in spheres of social welfare. This means relationships between social welfare, social work, social policy and human services more generally and feminism and feminist objectives as part of everyday life are the basic infrastructure of this book as well as its intellectual purpose.

The Positioning of Feminism

The initial, early prompting to write this book emerged from growing concerns about the apparent failures and fissures of feminism, the further we moved into the 21st century. As a feminist who recognised myself as a feminist as a very young woman, practised feminism throughout my daily life and pursued its application in analysis and research in my scholarship, I have had a sense that there may have been a shift away from some of the early aspirations of my local feminism, at least those that formed my emergence into feminism. This is not to suggest that feminism is not meant to be in a constant state of transformation or evolution, but it does suggest that for feminists and daughters of the second wave of feminism (late 1960s to the early 1990s), objectives for the overall project of feminism have changed, shifted, or failed. There is a difference between defining feminism and discussing one's *sense* of feminism as the definition relies on determinable and external arguments and evidence and one's sense of feminism is more complicated – it relates to how to live feminism, both as a sense of identity and as a framework for how to see, improve or change the world around you. This book is about both of those ways of seeing and doing feminisms. Once again, I acknowledge that this is my white feminist worldview, but it *is* inclusive of connections to my other passions for change which include countering the overwhelming consumption of the world's natural resources, to include in all political action the responsibility for our environment, our earth and the imperative to connect human need with sustainability. It is also inclusive of resistance to other 'isms' that oppress – racism, ageism, ableism – always aware that a core aspect of practice that resists is the capacity for emancipatory practice from both institutional and personal impositions.

It would be naïve to think that a body of thought and practice stands apart from cultural, political and marketised influences. Appropriations of feminism, for example, were achieved by creating commodified types of womanhood and girlhood that kept changing to keep pace with the broadest popularised social changes in attitudes about how women should be (Zeisler, 2016). The selling of feminine beauty as an element of women's 'emancipation' was explored by Michelle Lazar in her research on contemporary advertising's appropriation of choice and freedom in selling aids to being feminine as a 'right to be beautiful', as a fitting aspect of 'postfeminism' (2011, pp. 39–40).

The popularised commodification of feminism is an important point to make about white feminism's journey and how to be a feminist worker for social justice as it represents the constant pressure of popular notions of how to be a woman, which, due to their market or economic base, invariably impose exclusions based on gender, race, class, sexuality and/or ethnicity. It is important to see this wider context, a commodified world, that likes to use feminist ideas and even words but at the same time supports an anti-feminist agenda that works against social justice, because it is ever-present in every sphere of life. In fact, amid the rise of open right-wing, white-supremist views heralded by the election of President Trump (2017) in the USA, there is an extreme appropriation of some of feminism's achievements via the voice of women in that movement. Lana Lotkeff, a spokeswoman for alt-right women stated in a speech widely circulate via You Tube, that:

> *It was white women who got Trump elected and to be real edgy, it was also white women who got Hitler elected.* [And:]
>
> While feminists whine about the patriarchy and having another abortion (which, by the way, I'm OK with) we are raising the future of European countries.
>
> There are three important things for a woman, they are ingrained in our psyche and no matter how hard you try they will never be removed: beauty, family, home.
>
> *(Lotkeff, 2017)*

Although the Lotkeff example is extreme, it illustrates the complex capture of non-feminist identified women by asserting the collective empowerment of women so strongly promoted by feminism. She too appropriates feminism and is complicit with the idealised notion of how a woman should look (beauty) and behave (for family and the home). Conservative and 'alt-right' politics clings to traditional patriarchal ideals for women and eschews socially progressive movements that seek to gain equality for oppressed groups. However, on a more general level, this can be seen as a direct result of the power and success of the dominance of neoliberalism and the dominance of markets over social needs, but it also reflects the failure of feminism to entirely transform the world it had set out to change. On another level, it can be seen as the success of resistance to and a backlash against feminism or the successfully widespread circulation of the idea of a 'postfeminist' worldview adopted by some scholars and activists.

Postfeminism, a largely academic term, derived from 'evidence' in popular culture, has become a popularised concept in gender and cultural studies scholarship since the 1990s. It has also been propagated as part of the conservative backlash against feminism since the late 1970s in a deliberate negation of the women's movement (Hawkesworth, 2004, pp. 963–964). Although highly debatable, postfeminism refers to a proposition by some that much of the feminist agenda for equality (in the global North) has been achieved (women's equality in law for example) and that there is no specific need to maintain a feminist identified struggle. Also, as Gray and Boddy point out, it 'disempowers' feminism through a process of making it a redundant ideology of an early generation and instead values 'liberalizing processes that are connected to choice and diversity in domestic power – and introduce the white middle-class heterosexual woman as their symbol...' (2010, p. 383). This implies a double edge sword that promises the already privileged freedom of choice that has been distilled and propagated by free market capitalism but continues to determine needs and wants through marketing what 'a woman' wants.

Although postfeminism is not supported by contrary evidence of sustained women's movements across the world, nor strongly evident in research and scholarship related to social work, human development or social welfare, its basis in popular culture has had a significant impact on a generation of young women in the global North, whom may have otherwise been comfortable with identifying with feminism. From a personal perspective, this was strongly evident amongst social work and politics students that I taught from the late 1990s to around 2014, as at every opportunity I sought to gauge student reactions to feminism. The majority viewpoint was that it was distasteful to identify as a feminist because 'they are man-haters' or 'there is no need to be a feminist anymore'. However, after some inquiry into whether the women in the room had had experiences of sexism, there were realisations that the points of view held on that issue were indeed feminist and that sexism did require a feminist response. This process was not, however, enough to shift views on identifying as feminist as that identity had been well and truly tarnished via the anti-feminist backlash in politics and popular culture, not to mention the overriding of women's studies by the more ambiguous and not necessarily feminist field of 'gender studies'.

As Angela McRobbie points out 'postfeminism' was a process of 'disarticulation' where feminism became detached from other social justice movements. She saw it as:

> ...the objective of a new kind of gender power, which functions to foreclose on the possibility or likelihood of various expansive intersections of

intergenerational feminist transitions. Articulations are therefore reversed, broken off, and the idea of a new feminist imaginary becomes increasingly inconceivable. In social and cultural life there is instead a process of unpicking the seams of connection, forcing apart and dispersing subordinate social groups who might have possibly some common cause.

(McRobbie, 2009, p. 27)

There is a strong partnership between the disarticulation that socialist feminist McRobbie (2009) observed of 'postfeminism' and the rise and rise of neoliberalism. Both neoliberalism and 'postfeminism' engendered a force that devalued and negated collective action, or coming together as a form of social solidarity, on the basis that for individuals there is no need to do so – the neoliberal market supports individual choice, not societal choice. Therefore, in the postfeminist 'era', neoliberalism and postfeminism set out to prove that consumer choice is somehow gender equal or at least well catered for. Neoliberalism achieved this by commodifying what girls and women 'need' and selling and reproducing it through the indistinguishable products of mass media conveyed images of girl/woman celebrities, stars and products that make them individually aspirational and 'beautiful'.

However, in an unquestionably invigorating turn, my recent exploration and research about feminism have occurred over a period when there has been a visible, widespread revitalisation of public discourse about, and interest in, feminism and the emergence of a new generation of women and girls (and some men) identifying as feminists. Consequently, this book is not a straightforward exercise in reasserting feminism as a vitally important worldview. Rather, it is now a product of both the history of feminism and a lively, dynamic, contemporary environment of social and theoretical transformations. It is in this sense that I feel and see a re-emergence of feminism in the public sphere but also in research and scholarship. It is hoped that this book will add to the depth and quality of feminism's 'rebirth' as an essential framework for social welfare as well as for broad social change towards social justice and equality.

Practicing Feminism

Although what is meant by feminism will be teased out more fully in the following chapters, for now, it is enough to state that the idea that feminism is 'practiced' is central to its rationale and meaning. Feminism is about putting theory into practice; 'praxis' is theory in action. As bell hooks asserted, 'feminism is neither a lifestyle nor a ready-made identity or role one can step into' (1984, p. 26). Instead, feminism is the struggle to end sexist oppression, and out of that desire must come action; theory must become praxis. Hulko extends the concept of praxis by asserting that feminism also seeks to ensure 'that theory and practice are in conversation with one another' (2015, p. 69). From this point of view, my personal background, writing as I do as a white, older, heterosexual (cis gender), academic feminist, is less important than my commitment to feminism as a palette of theories that inform and interrogate the world and as a radical action-oriented movement that has always aimed to transform lives.

But this is not to suggest that I am not concerned with exploring my own positionality in relation to feminism. On the contrary, if I am to 'practice feminism', it is vital that I recognise my own privileges and interrogate my complicity in the oppression of others. As (now) a middle-class, educated white woman (from Australia), I have gained hugely from the achievements of liberal feminism; even my participation in higher education bears witness to the battles fought and won by earlier generations of (predominantly) white, middle-class women who sought, not to end sexist oppression, but to be treated as equals with men in their social class – particularly their fathers, brothers and husbands, the white patriarchy. Also, as a woman who first encountered feminism as a girl in the mid-1970s, I have benefited greatly from the opportunity to grow up and learn the personal and political lessons of feminism over a period of more than 40 years. I have also, of course, experienced and observed sexist discrimination and oppression, both within and outside the academy, in my working and personal life.

If I am 'practicing feminism' in writing this book, so too are you in reading the book, as you engage with its ideas and find yourself agreeing and disagreeing, connecting with, and rejecting its propositions and its claims. Drawing on the work of Michel de Certeau (1984), I invite readers to 'do feminism': to try it on for size, using it for their own purposes, personal, professional and political. Furthermore, I hope that in opening a view of social welfare practices to a feminist lens, theories and ideas that underpin them will become evident and central to effective practice for social justice and social change.

Social Welfare

The choice of 'social welfare' as the praxis location for this book was a carefully considered one. The longstanding writing and research on feminism and social work and feminism and social policy, is acknowledged (see Barrett, 1980; Brook and Davis, 1985; Blackburn, 1995; Cavanagh and Cree, 1996; Dale and Foster, 1986; Dominelli, 2002; Dominelli and McLeod, 1989; Hanmer and Statham, 1999; McIntosh, 2008; Pascall, 1997; Williams, 1989; Wilson, 1977), as well as the more recent literature, including Cree and Dean (2015), Phillips (2007, 2015), Phillips and Cree (2014), Wendt and Moulding (2016) and White (2006). Although this scholarship will form the backcloth for this book, wide theorising and research will also play an important role. This is reflected in the effort to try to do something different; something that is not restricted by the structures and organisational arrangements that the terms human services, social work and social policy inevitably throw up, nor the disciplinary constraint of situating it as a social work or social policy text. On the contrary, the aim is for this book to speak to, and engage with the ways that feminism is practised, as social welfare provision or struggles for welfare support, throughout the world, hence the decision to use what is presented as a broader, more inclusive concept of social welfare. This is not, of course, to assume that feminist practice is the same in all contexts; on the contrary, by locating feminism in different settings and countries, the diversity of feminism as a theory and practice will be highly evident.

Hence the term 'social welfare' is used in its most general sense to refer to, 'all social interventions intended to enhance or maintain the social functioning of human beings' (Dolgoff and Feldstein, 1999, p. 5). This is, however, a very apolitical definition of social welfare, which prompts some critical questions. For example, which human beings – all or some? Who decides? Why might some need help more than others? What is the political, economic, and social context that underpins this? This leads to the position that there must be a social justice imperative in social welfare. As Walter Lorenz writes, 'The term "social justice" has come to refer commonly to social policies and other rights-based initiatives that protect vulnerable and disadvantaged groups of national or global society from oppression, discrimination, and exclusion or that support them materially' (2014, p. 14). I will argue in this book that social justice and feminism must go together; that there cannot be social justice without attention to oppression based on gender identity. But at this stage, I simply repeat the global definition of social work as an example of that relationship:

> Social work is a practice-based profession and an academic discipline that promotes social change and development, social cohesion, and the empowerment and liberation of people. Principles of social justice, human rights, collective responsibility, and respect for diversities are central to social work. Underpinned by theories of social work, social sciences, humanities and indigenous knowledge, social work engages people and structures to address life challenges and enhance wellbeing.
>
> *(IFSW, 2014)*

As will be demonstrated in subsequent chapters of the book, feminism's engagement with social welfare is an essential aspect of work in a range of large and complex sites of welfare practice. This includes, for example, social work, international 'development', community services, income support, unemployment, nursing, community health, medical care (hospitals), housing, education, aged care, child and family support, disability services, mental health, reproductive care and advocacy, the justice system and community law. Much of the early social welfare provision in the global North was what might be described as 'gender blind'; it made a host of assumptions about gender roles and hierarchies and interrogated none of them. Yet social work was, and remains, overwhelmingly a women's profession (Orme, 2003), as are many of the other sites for social welfare. Social welfare is targeted at, and carried out by a largely female workforce, although men continue to dominate in positions of power within organisations (Pease, 2011). Social policy is also gendered throughout (Pascall, 1997), and the institutions of the welfare state bear witness to this. From the 16th century

British Poor Laws onwards, systems of social support have been founded on a 'man-as-breadwinner' and 'woman-as-helpmate-and-primary-carer' model. This was not challenged in any serious way by 'first wave' feminists, who, while fighting for the right to vote, often held to the notion that men should be providers and women should be homemakers, often comfortable in their educated class status. Thereafter, the evolution and establishment of the welfare state were founded on the concept of protecting citizens from the negative effects of the market and, eventually, the need to provide for basic human rights. Historically, the market largely excluded women from its direct benefits except at the most exploited levels of low-paid and unskilled labour. This would seem to suggest that women would have been a central focus for the welfare state and for research on the welfare state. However, even in the documentation of the history of the welfare state, as Gordon (1990) noted, much welfare state scholarship failed to recognise women's welfare as a core organising principle.

In the global North, it was not until the late 1960s and 1970s (the so-called 'second wave' of feminism) that women began to systematically confront the sexist ideology and practices within social welfare and, at the same time, work towards filling gaps in welfare support for women. Feminist scholars writing about poverty, social work, labour, childcare, education, incarceration and health as well as the welfare state were highly influential at that time. For example, Diana Pearce's (1978) coining of the term 'the feminisation of poverty' asserted the important relationship between women's low-paid work and their welfare needs, seeing it as a social policy problem distinct from men's welfare needs. At the same time, community-based women's refuges for women escaping domestic violence that sought to ensure physical protection from abuse and community-based women's health centres were established. These centres focused on reproductive rights and health and sexual assault services and were often established by women to support rape victims through legal, justice and health processes. Over time the women's movement pushed women's policy onto government agendas. The efforts of the women's movement (that also included pro-feminist men) encouraged governments to extend their responsibilities to fund the services that women activists had begun, and in doing so, extended the welfare state to address social issues such as domestic violence, child sexual abuse, reproductive and maternal health, and sexual assault. Such achievements came about in tandem with achievements in legislative change (including equal opportunity and anti-discrimination legislation, maternity leave policies, changes in the criminality of sexual assault, changes in laws related to marriage, property, divorce, etc.), political representation and education for women, reflecting the breadth and depth of feminist achievements in the global North.

More recent analyses and research on the welfare state has included voluminous feminist literature that has clearly established the extensive and sometimes contradictory relationships between women as consumers and providers of welfare. However, the real catch-up in welfare research has been the recognition of the predominance of women on or in need of welfare. This is often directly related to the intersection of gendered characteristics of being the main caregiver of children and other dependent family members, having less access to education and employment, particularly full-time employment, failing to have sufficient retirement savings, being victims of domestic violence or sexual assault and being at higher risk of poverty and homelessness. Moreover, women have been singled out, particularly within minority groups, and vilified by claims of welfare dependence. For example, in the USA, the issue of migration, particularly illegal migration of workers shifted from arguments about male migrants taking jobs from American citizens to immigrant women believed to be 'idle and welfare dependent mothers and inordinate breeders of dependents' (Chang, 2016, p. 4). As Chang (2016) further points out, the increased migration of women from developing countries relates not only to the economic crises of their home countries still suffering the wealth drain of having been colonised, but to the pull of employment as cheap, domestic, unskilled labour, particularly in the care industry. However, Ruiz et al. (2015), reported that in 2014 that the poverty rate of the poorest group of immigrant women, soul parent households, was equal to the number of non-immigrant poor sole parent women. It is also evident that migrant women to the USA are more likely to be employed legal migrants than male migrants. Across the world, views on migration are deeply intersected with views on race, class and gender and produce many stereotypes that must be countered via a social justice framework such as feminism.

It is also important to recognise and acknowledge that from my position, my global North perspective, I must counter stereotyped assumptions about women in the global South. It is important to avoid 'Orientalising' and generalising 'other' cultures and religious and ethnic identities (Said, 1978), avoid ideas that generalise the experiences of women. For example, as Elhum Haghighat points out the orientalist view of Islam as the 'secluder' and 'excluder' of women from the public domain, 'paints Middle Eastern women as submissive and powerless, living in a gender segregated world' (2010, p. 9). This is based on bundling all Islam as an undifferentiated group, when of course there are many types of practicing Muslims, just as there are diverse types of Christians. This is theoretically and practically vital from a feminist point of view.

Some Discussion of Terminology

Several key ideas and concepts have already been used in passing, and these will be central to the discussion and analyses throughout the book.

Waves of Feminism

A common and, in some ways, convenient way of thinking about, organising the history of and describing feminism is in terms of 'waves' (Phillips and Cree, 2014). Although the use of the wave metaphor has been criticised and debated for its tendency to create false distinctions and impose specific feminist identities on age cohorts (Chazan and Baldwin, 2017; Purvis, 2004) I do not intend it as a fixed set of categories or feminist identities. I agree that there is a fluidity in all feminist identities, which means there are no fixed, generational feminists but rather feminisms that became prominent at different points in time. Here I describe waves as a means of seeing how feminism was enacted and deployed in response to the various chronological contexts not as an identity of a feminist during those periods. I also acknowledge that is a predominantly global North metaphor and that there are no assumptions that feminisms developed and evolved in the same ways in the global South.

The term 'first wave' generally refers to the period from the mid-19th to the early 20th centuries when women in the global North (and some men) came together to confront a wide range of practices that affected the lives of women and children, including fighting for the promotion of equal contract and property rights for women; for women's right to vote; for legislation to protect women and girls from prostitution; for 'social purity'; for women's access to higher education and to the professions of medicine, law and accountancy. This was, in the main, an 'equal but different' kind of feminism, rooted in the sexual division of labour and it was also, in equal measure, classist, homophobic and, at times, racist. It was a product of privileged educated white women, reflective of the times when most women were denied education and any form of freedom of expression. As with every other period of women's resistance to domination, the reform agenda of the first wave was strenuously resisted by men in general but in the end won the mass support of women and key men in power to change the laws that denied equal citizenship rights and protection of women to a certain degree.

'Second wave' feminism can be characterised as the period from the early 1960s until the late 1980s, when the self-styled 'women's liberation movement' in the global North became involved in a range of activist campaigns: for women's reproductive rights and hence for legal access to abortions; for equal rights in employment and wages, education, public and private lives; against rape and domestic violence; against pornography and prostitution; against sexism in the media; against work discrimination; against sexual harassment; against unequal rights to property; and uneven representation in politics. Second-wave feminism saw individual, sexual, social, and political inequalities as inevitably interlinked; 'the personal is political' was a popular radical feminist slogan. Although not limited to heteronormativity, it was within this political stance that specific intimate relationships with men were challenged, related to family roles, expectations and constraints of marriage and sexual equality. Strong, divergent theoretical and activist strands of feminism emerged in this period and most endure in some form today, including radical, liberal, socialist, black, separatist, and cultural feminisms. There were many challenges to second-wave feminism, but none greater than the critique of its universalising tendency of 'women' and its dominant white, Western middle-class voice that was not seen to represent women from diverse racial, cultural, and ethnic backgrounds.

Reflecting a widespread, postmodern theoretical turn away from structuralism in the 1990s, a new conceptualisation of feminism came to the fore, challenging the 'grand narratives' of second-wave feminism (Mani, 2013). This meant an objection to the overarching concept of patriarchy and any sense of a shared oppression by all women, which was seen as a failed universalisation of women's individual experiences as women. 'Third wave' feminists had no problem with the notion that there might be different feminisms, and that gender was something, as Judith Butler argued, that was 'performed', not innate (Butler, 1990). Meanwhile, oppression based on gender was understood as something that intersected with other areas of oppression, including those of 'race' and ethnicity, age, social class, and disability. Broadly, third-wave feminism included important assertions of Southern feminism including 'third world' feminism, postcolonial feminism and African 'womanism'. 'Fourth-wave' feminism has taken the third-wave project even further, as social media opened up significant spaces for feminist debates and resistance; commentators such as Baumgardner (2011) go so far as to argue that fourth-wave feminism was born in 2008 on social media. Unpacking the direction of the fourth wave, Munro (2013) suggests that the new social media-based feminism is intolerant of all 'isms' and inclusive of diverse sexualities and cultures. It reflects the popularity of intersectionality as a theoretical frame for analysis and seeks to contest the idea of feminists as 'man-hating' or 'bra burning' (reacting to the backlash against feminism's stereotyping of feminists by what was seen as the most confronting aspects of feminist action and identity). Instead, fourth-wave feminism appears to seek an equality that demobilises the power of one gender over another and shames sexist and violent behaviour wherever it is found (see also Cochrane, 2013).

In a cross-national study between Australia and Germany that I conducted with a German colleague in 2016, which sought to explore feminist identity amongst feminist activists working in women's NGOs or on women's programs, there was very little identification with the concept of a fourth wave of feminism. In fact, when asked about understanding of the waves of feminism, most of the research participants did not recognise waves as valuable distinctions, although younger women were clearly critical or even hostile about the dominance of second wavers and what were seen as limited ideas of feminism.

This has been an abbreviated journey through the waves of feminism. But the subject cannot end here. Firstly, it is important to acknowledge that the waves of feminism do not actually exist – they are abstract – and feminists do not all fit neatly into one or another wave. On the contrary, it is highly likely that fourth-wave feminists may (consciously and unconsciously) draw on second-wave ideas, just as the distinction between third and fourth waves may be more transparent than real. For example, feminists in the second wave in the United Kingdom deliberately claimed their turf as feminists by looking back to the suffragette movement of the late nineteenth and early 20th centuries for inspiration. But in doing so, they ignored (and at times dismissed) the struggles and achievements of their mothers' generation; women whose activism had found its place during the

Second World War through to the creation of a post-war welfare state. If feminism's waves are abstract, however, this does not negate the usefulness of the idea. On the contrary, the notion of waves offers a useful analytical tool; a way of ordering the experience of feminism within the context of periods of social change. Further, this sense of generational connectedness between the waves is contrary to McRobbie's concerns about the ruptures of feminism and her expressed concern about postfeminism's capacity to 'foreclose on the possibility or likelihood of various expansive intersections of intergenerational feminist transitions' (2009, p. 27). This is because at the time of writing this book there is clearly a greater enthusiasm for reclaiming many aspects of earlier feminist legacies for strategic action and social change, as well as engagement and optimism about its continually evolving future and role. Consequently, I will return to the prospects and characteristics of the fourth wave in the concluding chapter of this book.

Global North, South and West

Another concept that is used in this book is the idea of a global North and global South. There have been many ways of distinguishing between countries in recent years, including North/South, West/East, minority/majority, developed/ developing, industrialised/industrialising and rich/poor, and I have been challenged by which terms might be most useful for analytical purposes. It is acknowledged that all these terms are imperfect; they inevitably forefront certain aspects of structural inequality and miss out on others. In the end, however, the global North/global South terminology will be used because it offers a distinction based not only on geography or population size or on an idea of what social 'progress' might mean. On the contrary, the global North/global South distinction highlights the complex and interconnecting economic, political and hegemonic theoretical power held by countries that are currently referred to as the North as compared with those that are technically in the South (Willis, 2010). The distinction is a fluid one, because countries like Australia, although geographically in the South, are grouped with Northern countries, based on its wealth, power through political alliances and British colonial status. Nevertheless, it is seen as the most efficient way of grasping quickly the difference between the powerful Northern countries, which are generally wealthier, have been industrialised for some time and were the colonisers, and continue to exert most political power (although now challenged by superpower countries like China and India) and countries in the global South, which have held less power and importantly, are likely to be poorer economically in comparison to those in the North. However, at times the term Western as an alternative to Northern, may be applied because this notion helpfully flags Eurocentrism, reminding us of the constructed dichotomies between the dominant, hegemonic West, and the object of 'otherness', the East. It is also commonly applied to separate cultural perceptions and practices within feminism but must be recognised for its loaded differentiation in historical terms, as will be discussed more fully in Chapter 2.

Women and Feminism

Feminism has been criticised, at various points in time, for seeming to essential-ise women: in effect, to assume that there is one category 'woman' and that all women's needs, and experiences are the same. This is a critical point for the rela-tionship between white feminists and women of colour, especially in the failure of white feminists to examine their own white race privilege in their engage-ment with women of colour (Moreton-Robinson, 2020). Feminists have also been criticised for seeming to treat all men as if they are the same, that is, most commonly as oppressors, perpetrators of violence and rapists. These accusations have been made by critics from both within and outside the women's movement and were heard most loudly in the 1990s with what has been described as a back-lash against feminism (see Faludi, 1991). It is not my intention to rehearse these arguments again in this book. Rather, it is my assertion that there is not one single way of practicing feminism, just as there is not a single category 'woman'. As the practice examples in this book will illuminate, women from different classes, gender alignment, ethnicities, countries, ages, and abilities have taken on feminist causes and fought against sex and gender oppression wherever they have encountered it. This does not, and, I believe, cannot, mean that they were always aware of, or aligned to, other oppressions or experiences. Scholars have identified versions of feminism from the conservative right through to the radical left, and individual feminists may have had more in common with others of their own race, class, ethnicity, or sexuality than with other self-identifying feminists at moments in history. We are always, at the end of the day, creatures of our time – of the available knowledge and experience and the total of our under-standing at the time, impartial and incomplete as this inevitably is. Because of this, there will always be conflict and disagreement between us about how to practice feminism, as is demonstrated in the current debates between trans and 'cisgender' women regarding the place of sex and gender within feminism and within society (Aultman, 2014). I will not attempt to resolve any of these issues. Rather, I will argue that by examining them in more depth, through the exam-ples of praxis, we may get close to understanding what it means to practice fem-inism in social welfare today.

Outline of Following Chapters

In Chapter 2, I take a broad perspective of how feminism has been placed and continues to operate on the global social policy agenda. Global feminism is evident in institutional social policy responses to global social problems. This chapter explores the impact of gender equality policies in both Northern and Southern countries. It also raises key questions such as: Why hasn't feminism brought about gender equality globally? Where does feminism fit with ideas of human rights and social justice, and with an individualised, privatised con-sumer culture? What has the impact of neoliberal dominance been on feminism, particularly in rich Western democracies? This chapter includes insights from African feminist practitioners to demonstrate the diversity of how feminism is interpreted and practiced depending on the key intersections of race, class and gender as well as the critical aspect of 'nation' or national context.

Chapter 3 explores one of the most important social policy issues for feminists. This chapter focuses on domestic violence, discussing feminism's contribution to theory, policy and practice around domestic violence. Given how long domestic or family violence has been on feminist agendas, it is not surprising that this is an area of feminist practise that has also faced inner challenges about how feminist practise has addressed and intervened on both a service or practice level and at a policy level. Therefore, the chapter also problematises feminisms' relationships to domestic violence. Key questions are raised and discussed. Why is there still such violence against women worldwide? Is a new analysis of power and domination needed?

Chapter 4 focuses on motherhood, birthing rights, maternal agency, maternal deaths, obstetric violence and the loss of a baby. Although the term motherhood is used, the contemporary capacity for transgender men to bear children is recognised and the specific challenges faced by transgender birth parents are acknowledged. The chapter also highlights how social welfare in motherhood is problematised in how mothers are constructed as consumers, as the producer of bloodlines, as a unit of reproduction and in a role under intense scrutiny and expectations. The global perspective explored in this chapter demonstrates that women as mothers undergo specific exploitations and oppressions because of their capacity to reproduce and their welfare is often undermined by failures in access to basic human rights as maternal and mother rights. Chapter 5, Reproductive Justice, Rights and Welfare, the Role of Feminist Practice, extends the focus on the complexities of social welfare related to reproduction, exploring women's agency over their bodies and societal, religious, cultural, market and political impositions on the role of women as reproductive units. The chapter begins with an examination of social welfare related to experiences of menstruation, and its cultural and economic consequences. By looking at abortion and assisted reproduction as an important 'technologies' for self-determining when, whether or how to have a child and even the capacity to select the gender of a child, are also part of this discussion. As are the news ways that motherhood has become commodified through commercial, inter-country surrogacy.

In Chapter 6, a discussion of feminism and working with older people is presented as an increasingly important component of social welfare across the world as populations are rapidly ageing. As women have outlived men traditionally by some years, the older and very old population must be a focus for feminist practice. This involves addressing many ageist oppressions that place women (and people with minority sexual and cultural identities) in particularly disempowered circumstances as they begin to grow old and become very old in their communities. Areas of welfare support for older women are related to higher risks of poverty and homelessness due to a life course that has left them without resources. The political economy for older women relates, across all countries, to deeply entrenched economic subordination via lack of access to education and precarious employment, patriarchal roles that have excluded them from independent wealth accumulation, social and political exclusion, the burden of care and so on. In response to this, this chapter explores what an emancipatory practice with older people would look like? How can feminism help to challenge neoliberal ideals of anti-dependency and increasing institutionalisation?

Chapter 7 focuses on feminist practice and perspectives on the law and the criminal justice system.

This chapter explores the specific impositions of the law on women and the policing of populations and behaviours. Women's experiences of imprisonment and intersections with their roles as carers and mothers as well as the impact of poverty as a key cause of incarceration arise in this chapter. Also, the injustice of a criminal justice system that has been steeped in patriarchal laws that have privileged men's prerogatives in relation to issues of domestic violence, and sexual assault is a key area examined as it has deep effects on women's welfare. This chapter also returns to issues of reproductive justice in exploring how laws have been created and imposed to control women, particularly in relation to abortion.

Chapter 8 pulls many ideas in this book together and, to be forward looking, it focuses on an understanding of the fourth wave and how it strengthens feminist practice in welfare. In this final chapter of the book, the central characteristics that appear to establish a distinct fourth-wave feminism are explored. The discussion highlights the most repeated aspects of fourth-wave identity: intersectionality and gender inclusivity. The discussion centres on two things, first the counterpoints and shifts that fourth-wave feminists appear to be demanding of earlier-wave identity feminists. The fusing of intersectionality as a type of feminism is central within the voices of self-defined fourth wavers and is discussed in relation to earlier feminist engagement with this important lens for action and analysis. The second key characteristic and distinctiveness of the fourth wave is the issue of acting in the interests of all genders and the challenge to move beyond the 'cis-gender' woman focus of earlier waves of feminism. This is a touchpoint for the fourth wave that has resulted in a lively dispute amongst feminists. However, the major intent of this discussion is to examine how feminist practice engages and supports social welfare now and into the future.

Conclusion

There is one 'big idea' at the heart of this book: that social welfare needs to be explored and responded to through a feminist lens. Without such a perspective, the idea of the 'personal is political' will be missed, as will gendered structures of inequality and oppression. But the feminism that is embraced is not a simplistic, essentialist one; instead, it is highly related to context. So, I acknowledge both the strengths and conflicts within feminism; the complexities and the contradictions that have led to criticisms from both within and outside feminist discourse.

This is not a comprehensive analysis of the relationship between and experiences of feminist practice and social welfare, rather I have chosen several practice settings and set out to tell a story of feminism's engagement with, and impact on theory, policy, and practice in each – in other words, I explore what it means to 'practice feminism' from a globally informed perspective. In doing so, I aim to add to the agenda for feminist social welfare policy responses and feminist practice for social justice into the future.

References

Aultman, B. (2014) Cisgender. *Transgender Studies Quarterly*, 1 (1–2), 61–62.

Barrett, M. (1980) *Women's Oppression Today Problems in Marxist Feminist Analysis*. London: Verso.

Baumgardner, J. (2011) Is there a fourth Wave? Does it matter? From the book *F'em Goo Goo, Gaga and Some Thoughts on Balls*. https://www.feminist.com/resources/artspeech/genwom/baumgardner2011.html.

Blackburn, S. (1995) How useful are feminist theories of the welfare state? *Women's History Review*, 4 (3), 369–394.

Brook, E. and Davis, A. (1985) *Women, the Family, and Social Work*. London; New York: Tavistock Publications.

Butler, J. (1990) *Gender Trouble*. London: Routledge.

Cavanagh, K. and Cree, V. (eds) (1996) *Working with Men, Feminism and Social Work*. London: Routledge.

Chang, G. (2016) *Disposable Domestics: Immigrant Women Workers in the Global Economy* (2nd ed.). Chicago, IL: Haymarket Books.

Chazan, M. and Baldwin, M. (2016) Understanding the complexities of contemporary feminist activism. *Feminist Formations*, 28 (3), 70–94.

Cochrane, K. (2013) The fourth wave of feminism: Meet the rebel women. *The Guardian*, Wednesday, December 11, 05.55 AEDT. https://www.theguardian.com/world/2013/dec/10/fourth-wave-feminism-rebel-women.

Cree, V.E. and Dean, J.S. (2015) Exploring social work students' attitudes towards feminism: Opening up conversations. *Social Work Education*, 34 (8), 903–920.

Dale, J. and Foster, P. (1986) *Feminists and State Welfare*. London; Boston, MA: Routledge & Kegan Paul.

de Certeau, M. (1984) *The Practice of Everyday Life*. Berkeley: University of California Press.

Dolgoff, R. and Feldstein, D. (1999) *Understanding Social Welfare* (5th ed.). Boston, MA: Allyn and Bacon.

Dominelli, L. (2002) *Feminist Social Work Theory and Practice*. Basingstoke: Palgrave.

Dominelli, L. and McLeod, E. (1989) *Feminist Social Work*. Basingstoke: Macmillan.

Hanmer, J. and Statham, D. (1999) *Women and Social Work: Towards a Woman Centred Practice* (2nd ed.). Basingstoke: Macmillan.

Eyadat, Z. (2013) Islamic feminism: Roots, development and policies. *Global Policy*, 4 (4), 359–368.

Faludi, S. (1991) *Backlash: The Undeclared War against American Women* (1st ed.). New York: Crown Publishing.

Gordon, L. (1990) The welfare state: Towards a socialist-feminist perspective. *Socialist Register*, 26, 171–200.

Gray, M. and Boddy, J. (2010) Making sense of the waves: Wipeout or still riding high? *Affilia: Journal of Women and Social Work*, 25 (4), 368–389.

Gunew, S. (1990) Feminist knowledge, critique and construct. In S. Gunew (ed.) *Feminist Knowledge, Critique and Construct*. London: Routledge, 13–35.

Haghighat, E. (2010) *Women in the Middle East and Africa, Change and Continuity*. New York: Palgrave Macmillan.

Hawkesworth, M. (2004) The semiotics of premature burial: Feminism in a postfeminist age. *Signs: Journal of Women in Culture and Society*, 29 (4), 961–985.

hooks, bell. (1984) *Feminist Theory: From Margin to Center*. Cambridge, MA: South End Press.

Hulko, W. (2015) Operationalizing intersectionality in feminist social work research: Reflections and techniques from research with equity-seeking groups. In S. Wahab, B. Anderson-Nathe and C. Gringeri (eds) *Feminisms in Social Work Research: Promise and Possibilities for Justice-based Knowledge*. Abingdon; New York: Routledge, 6989.

IFSW (International Federation of Social Work) (2014) *Global Definition of the Social Work Profession*. http://ifsw.org/policies/definition-of-social-work/.

Lazar, M. (2011) The right to be beautiful: Postfeminist identity and consumer beauty advertising. In R. Gill and C. Schaff (eds) *New Femininities, Postfeminism, Neoliberalism and Subjectivity*. Basingstoke; New York: Palgrave Macmillan, 37–51.

Lombardo, E. and Verloo, M.M. (2009) Contentious citizenship: Feminist debates and practices and European challenges. *Feminist Review*, 92 (1), 108–128.

Lorenze, W. (2014) The emergence of social justice in the West. In M. Reisch (ed.) *The Routledge International Handbook of Social Justice*. Oxon; New York: Routledge, 14–26.

Lotkeff, L. (2017) How the Left is betraying women. *Identitarian Ideas IX*. https://www.youtube.com/watch?v=BjnH99slHmE.

Mani, K. (2013) *The Integral Nature of Things: Critical Reflections on the Present*. New Delhi: Routledge.

McIntosh, M. (2008) Feminism and social policy. *Critical Social Policy*, 1 (1), 32–42.

McRobbie, A. (ed.) (2009) *The Aftermath of Feminism*. London; Thousand Oaks; New Delhi: SAGE Publications.

Morton-Robinson, A. (2000) *Talkin' Up to the White Woman: Aboriginal Women and Feminism*. St Lucia: University of Queensland Press.

Munro, E. (2013) Feminism: A fourth wave? *Political Insight*. London: The Political Studies Association (PSA). http://www.psa.ac.uk/insight-plus/feminism-fourth-wave.

Orme, J. (2003) It's feminist because I say so!: Feminism, social work and critical practice in the UK. *Qualitative Social Work*, 2, 131–154.

Pascall, G. (1997) *Social Policy: A New Feminist Analysis*. London; New York: Routledge.

Pearce, D. (1978) The feminization of poverty: Women, work and welfare. *Urban and Social Change Review*, 11 (1 & 2), 28–36.

Pease, B. (2011) Men in social work: Challenging or reproducing an unequal gender regime? *Affilia*, 26 (4), 406–418.

Phillips, R. (2007) The place of feminism in contemporary social work education in Australia. *Advances in Social Work and Welfare Education*, 9 (1), 54–68.

Phillips, R. (2015) How 'empowerment' may miss its mark: Gender equality policies and how they are understood in women's NGOs. *Voluntas: International Journal of Voluntary and Nonprofit Organizations*, 26 (4), 1122–1142.

Phillips, R. and Cree, V.E. (2014) What does the 'fourth wave' mean for teaching feminism in Twenty-first century social work? *Social Work Education: The International Journal*, 33 (7), 930–943.

Purvis, J. (2004) Girls and women together in the third wave: Embracing the challenges of intergenerational feminism(s). *NWSA Journal*, 16 (3), 93–123.

Ramirez, R. (2007) Race, tribal nation, and gender, a nativist feminist approach to belonging. *Meridians: Feminism, Race, Transnationalism*, 7 (20), 22–40.

Ruiz, A.G., Zong, J. and Batalova, J. (2015) *Immigrant Women in the United States*. Washington, DC: Migration Policy Institute. http://www.migrationpolicy.org/article/immigrant-women-united-states#Employment%20and%20Occupations.

Safi, M. (2020) All the people: What happens if humanity's ranks start to shrink? *The Guardian*, Saturday, July 25, 2020, 14.00 AEST. https://www.theguardian.com/world/2020/jul/25/all-the-people-what-happens-if-humanitys-ranks-start-to-shrink.

Said, E. (1978) *Orientalism*. London: Routledge & Kegan Paul.

Shaw, C.M. (2015) *Women and Power in Zimbabwe, Promises of Feminism*. Champaign: University of Illinois Press.

Stanley, L. (ed.) (1990) *Feminist Praxis: Research, Theory and Epistemology in Feminist Research*. London: Routledge.

Tedmanson, D. and Fejo-King, C. (2016) Talking up and listening well, dismantling whiteness and building reflexivity. In S. Wendt and N. Moulding (eds) *Contemporary Feminism in Social Work Practice* (1st ed.). London: Routledge, 149–165.

Vollset, S.E., Goren, E., Yuan, C., Cao, J., Smith, A.E., Hsiao, T., et al. (2020) Fertility, mortality, migration, and population scenarios for 195 countries and territories from 2017 to 2100: A forecasting analysis for the Global Burden of Disease Study. *The Lancet*, 396 (10258), 1285–1306. https://www.thelancet.com/journals/lancet/article/PIIS0140-6736(20)30677-2/fulltext.

Wendt, S. and Moulding, N. (eds) (2016) *Contemporary Feminism in Social Work Practice*. London: Routledge.

White, V. (2006) *The State of Feminist Social Work*. London: Routledge.

Williams, F. (1989) *Social Policy: A Critical Introduction: Issues of Race, Gender and Class*. Cambridge: Polity Press.

Willis, K. (2010) *Theories and Practices of Development* (2nd ed.). London; New York: Routledge.

Wilson, E. (1977) *Women and the Welfare State*. London: Tavistock.

Zeisler, A. (2016) *We Were Feminists Once, from Riot Grrrl to CoverGirl, the Buying and Selling of a Political Movement*. New York: Public Affairs.

2

GLOBAL FEMINISM, GLOBAL SOCIAL POLICY AND SOCIAL WELFARE

Introduction

To establish the world-wide context of feminist practice, this chapter explores international engagement with and perspectives on feminism and the impact of feminist practice across the world, with a particular focus on the diversity of feminisms, feminist thought and praxis and its relation to global social policy and social welfare. I also discuss globally promoted gender-equality policies, exploring why feminism hasn't brought about gender equality globally. Other implicit questions in this chapter and throughout this book are: What is the role of women's/feminist NGOs in pursuing gender equality? Where does feminism fit with ideas of human rights and social justice, and with an individualised, privatised consumer culture? What has the impact of neoliberal dominance been on feminism, particularly in the wealthy global North?

As discussed in the introduction to this book, there has been an explosion of interest in feminism in recent years. This has been, witnessed in academic writing across a range of disciplines (including Bell et al., 2019; Bowden and Mummery, 2009; David, 2014; Dillon, 2007; Gillis et al., 2007; Gray and Boddy, 2010; Marcos and Waller, 2016; McRobbie, 2009, 2015; Mohanty, 2003; Phipps, 2020; Rottenberg, 2014; Shaw, 2015; Simões et al., 2021; Walby, 2011) and in digital and analogue popular media. It has also been demonstrated in local and global gender equality policies and research (OECD, 2020; UNMDGs, 2013; UNSDGs, 2022; UN Women, 2015; WHO, 2021; World Economic Forum, 2021) and in initiatives at local and global levels that seek to address all the many issues and concerns that are at the heart of feminism. The term feminism is also appearing more often than previously in global goals, for example the World Health Organisation along with the United Nations, released a series of research papers on 'Women's Health and Gender Inequalities' which articulated an agenda

DOI: 10.4324/9781315625188-2

that included 'investing in feminist movements, which have been instrumental in fostering progressive changes towards gender equality' and 'ensuring women's and feminist leadership in governments, health and development agencies, and other global organizations' (WHO, 2021).

Social media has also opened significant spaces for the resurgence of feminist debates and resistances, and it has been argued that social media or the Internet is the birthplace of 'fourth wave' feminism (Baumgardner, 2011; Leupold, 2010; Phillips and Cree, 2014). Of course, from a global North perspective a growth in interest in feminism has been most visibly white feminism and has been popularised through the dominance of neoliberal feminism in response to specific public issues, emanating mostly from the USA. I refer here to the '#MeToo' movement and the anti-Trump feminist (pink hats) movement. As Phipps (2020) points out, although the #MeToo movement was initiated by an African American feminist, it was popularised via the prominence of celebrity of white women actors and its focus on 'Me' became a parallel to the ideology of individualist neoliberalism, enabling it to become popularised in hegemonic global North popular media. Despite this, the fight against sexism at the core of the movement became a catch call for feminist action across the world, including the global South. Phipps (2020) also points out that despite the capacity of white feminism to dominate through its powerful national vehicles, it is not definitive of feminism. This book relies on the acknowledgement, recognition and deference to the diversity of feminist practice, identities and contexts despite my obvious place as a white feminist.

As part of the renewed public interest in feminism across the world, extensive blogs, Facebook pages, Twitter campaigns, TikTok posts and websites are restating the objectives and demands of broad feminist movements and agendas today. One key aspect of the use of digital communications as feminist action and communication is the intensification of global networks, national and cross-national collaboration and shared political goals and objectives. However, in a global study I conducted from 2011 to 2013, which, in part, explored how women's NGOs defined their feminism and feminist activism, it was found that there is much diversity in understandings and theories of feminism, which related to diverse political theories and identities, key social issues within local contexts, as well as political and economic factors within states and communities (Phillips, 2015). The diversity of feminism as theory, feminist identity and feminist practice, combined as praxis, is at the heart of both its appeal as a social movement and its internal and external contestations. Therefore, in keeping with the focus of this book and in asserting some broad generalisations about feminism across the world, it is useful to clarify how feminism can be viewed as a practice.

One way of viewing feminist practice is as radical action in pursuit of social justice and equality. Eschle and Maiguashca, as a part of a critical analysis of socialist feminist critiques of contemporary feminism, suggest that *radical* social action can be seen as a 'quest for a particular kind of social change, namely a transformation of systemic power relations perceived to sustain ongoing injustices' and is linked to political projects (2014, p. 646). They further point out that this may occur incrementally, abruptly or in a slow evolutionary process and that what matters in their definition of radical action is 'not the concrete strategy through which change is achieved, but the scope of the ambition behind it' (Eschle and Maiguashca, 2014, p. 646). What is clear when examining how feminism is practiced across the world is the breadth and scope of its ambitions and how persistent the core objectives of emancipation and equality are despite its extremely diverse contexts. Eschle and Maiguashca's (2014) definition of radical social action is a highly applicable concept for examining feminism as a practice across the world because it encapsulates what is generalisable about all feminist practice, a quest for a transformation of systemic power relations that are seen to sustain ongoing injustices or oppression. Depending on the context and the capacities at hand, this can occur at an interpersonal level, a community level, a national level or at an international level.

This chapter initially focuses on why and how feminism is important across the world, whilst also unpacking what feminist practice is, it then focuses on the role of women's/feminist NGOs and explores how the practice of feminism has transformed global social policy responses to key social issues. It then focuses on the relationships between feminist practice and social welfare in the global context as well as arguing for feminist approaches to global social policy.

Background: Feminisms across the World

When contemporary feminism emerged as a social change movement for equality across the world, albeit predominantly in 'the North', either as driven by suffragettes in the first wave of the women's movement or by those of the more recent second or third waves, activists had many objectives and faced many challenges to achieving them. However, the objectives pursued by feminist activists had few limits, they were and are deeply personal and private, and widely public and political. As a result, women's various struggles for equality have been played out in many sites of daily life and within institutions as well as in the production, formation and reformation of knowledge and thought. Feminism has a long history that is not simply attached to contemporary articulations or theories of feminism or even the well-defined Western notion of 'waves' of feminism because, as a form of action and resistance and often left out of historiographies, it has been intrinsic to the way women have been positioned in all civilisations, religions and cultures across most of recorded history.

In their introduction to *New French Feminisms*, Marks and De Courtivron (1980) included an abbreviated genealogy of the history of feminism in France. This account of history is based on an important premise for why feminism existed:

> Feminism owes its existence to the universality of misogyny, gynophobia, androcentrism, and heterosexism. Feminism exists because women are,

and have been, everywhere oppressed at every level of exchange from the simplest social intercourse to the most elaborate discourse. Whatever the origins of this oppression – biological, economic, psychological, linguistic, ontological, political, or some combination of these – a polarity of opposites based on sexual analogy organizes our language and through it directs our manner of perceiving the world.

(Marks and De Courtivan, 1980, p. 4)

To demonstrate how women have been defined in relation to men, Marks and De Courtivan's (1980) account of the history of feminism in France began as early as the year 496. At this time early Catholicism was structured as a church that asserted and reinforced the social inferiority of women, subsequently, in the early 6th century the church ensured that women could not inherit land, by the 10th century women were established by the church as the major source of evil, excluded from monarchical rule and, from the mid-13th century, persecuted as witches, burnt at the stake for independence and outstanding action (Joan of Arc), dispossessed of land and so on (Marks and De Courtivan, 1980, pp. 10–27). However, throughout French history, there is also evidence of a persistent debate about women's equality. Such writings were mostly by enlightened men until the Renaissance when women of means, with access to education, began to publish works that argued against the repression and denigration of women's minds and later poor women asserted their voice by demonstrating in solidarity and collective action through revolution and demands for food security. Two important and persistent aspects of feminism that emerged from this very abbreviated story of French history were the distinct relationships between gender and class in struggles for equality and the persistence of women resisting oppressions.

What happened in French history was of course a set of struggles that were duplicated in other countries and communities throughout time and with various levels of success and were not restricted to the global North. As Raewyn Connell (2015) observed in a discussion of the production of feminist knowledge from the global South, there is a long history of feminist action within diverse cultures. Connell described the 'rich history of thought and debate about gender equality' that can be traced to 17th century Mexico and later in the late 19th and early 20th centuries when women such as Aisha Taymour in Egypt, author of 'The Mirror of Contemplating Affairs' (1892) analysed concerns about women in Qur'anic texts and Raden Adjeng Kartini, author of 'Letters of a Javanese Princess' (1911) who in her writing asserted feminist principles, seeking to free herself from the traditional expectations of a young woman of her time and how her protestations inspired generations of Indonesian feminists (2015, p. 54). What is also evident is that countries that are currently blatantly repressive of women and feminism, have had prior, more emancipated political histories where feminists were openly present and fighting for equality such as 1920s China and late 19th century Egypt (Connell, 2015; Eyadat, 2013). However, what is so profound for us now, considering how long women's resistance to oppression and struggles for emancipation have gone on, is the on-going need for and nature of similar struggles right through to the 21st century, and no doubt, into the future.

Contemporary feminism in France, in 2016, for example, was similarly controversial as in most large, rich Western countries, and in recent years has emerged again in popular debate. Issues that bring feminism into the public domain in the present seem universal and form elements of a well-rehearsed set of conflicts and debates or struggles about power and domination. This is played out at various social levels and via the entire spectrum of media. It is inclusive of celebrities identifying as feminists, or denying feminist identity, through grassroots campaigns for women's rights to ethnic or religious freedoms. Revised and new considerations for feminism have appeared as the intersectionality of race, diversity in gender identity, age, disability and faith have become both core challenges to and core causes for much feminist action.

However feminism, as a sum of all its parts, has had a history of institutional as well as social and community achievements and continues to influence key decisions on social policies, for example in April 2016, the French National Assembly adopted a Nordic response to prostitution (already applied in five countries) by recognising prostitution and the linked trafficking of women, as a form of violence against women, and decided to criminalise the purchase of sex in France, shifting the blame from sex workers (mostly women) to the people who buy sex (mostly men) and offering financial assistance for sex-workers to find different work (Huffington Post, 2016). This legislation was, however, equally critiqued by some feminists who align themselves with a free choice view of sex work. They see the legislation as an oppression of sex workers' choice to sell their bodies, highlighting how feminism, through the intrinsic attempts to avoid universalising the experiences of women and the need to embrace diversity and intersectionality, creates its own, often long-running, divisions.

The same debate was also highlighted in Australia when a group of women convened the 'first' abolitionist conference to advocate for a similar legal model as the Nordic Model in Australian laws on prostitution. In an article on a feminist news website 'Feminist Current', it reported attempts by a pro-sex work advocacy group in Australia to shut down the conference (Murphy, 2016). The conference entitled '*The World's Oldest Oppression*' included several 'survivors' of prostitution and sex trafficking who spoke in favour of abolishing prostitution. The group that campaigned against the conference, using virulent social media threats, was a sex worker advocacy group with a vocal opposition to the Nordic model of legislation. Regardless of how the group positioned itself in relation to feminism, there are feminist arguments to support women sex workers and the choice to be part of the pornography industry, which has often been seen as similarly exploitative and oppressive of women by major radical feminist scholar/activists, including Barry (1979, 1995), MacKinnon (1985) and Dworkin (1987, 1993). As discussed in Chapter 1, feminisms are characterised by diverse and sometimes oppositional politics and have constantly evolved according to historical, political, social and economic contexts.

What is also evident, however, is that within specific groups or national and ethnic identities, organic forms of feminism have emerged, demonstrating the capacity for feminist practice to take place in diverse contexts. For example, as Eyadat explains, despite a possible Western feminist view that may see Islam and feminism as contradictory, Islamic feminism was heavily influenced by dominant Western feminisms from the 1970s to the 1990s and is viewed as an 'expression of enlightenment and reconciliation between religious beliefs and egalitarianism' (2013, p. 359). Eyadat also suggests that with support from Western feminists and by placing Islamic feminism within a human rights framework, given the broader democracy movement of the Arab Spring, the Arab world is well positioned to promote Islamic feminism within wider Arab society (2013, p. 359). However, she pointed out that there is a wide diversity within Arab feminism that includes a reaction to Western feminism as a re-colonising force. For example, the widespread adoption of the headscarf and other forms of traditional dress is seen as a reaction to hegemonic Western feminist views of Islam's oppression of women:

> The diversity of Islamic feminism means that it does not necessitate certain styles of clothing, but the wide-spread donning of more conservative garb exhibits the rise in women's self-assertion and women's rights, a measure against societal and gender norms. In direct opposition to a foreign brand of feminism, the women of Egypt and the majority of women across the entire Arab world demonstrated that their choices were their own, rather than embracing the cultural values of another society.
>
> *(Eyadat, 2013, p. 362)*

Due to highly politicised public discussions of Islam arising from extremist Islamic terrorism across many parts of the world, tensions have also arisen around the question of just how feminist Islamic women can be. This has been a particular focus in Western countries where Muslim minority women engage in public debate arguing that Islam can be feminist (Abdel-Magied, 2017; Carland, 2017; Malik, 2017).

Although Eyadat's (2013) proposition of a self-defined feminist identity for Arab women must be recognised and supported from a feminist, social justice perspective, challenges that are the same for most formal religions arise for Western feminists, especially for second-wave feminists. Most formal religions traditionally positioned women as secondary to men within the practices and tenets of the religion. This is a complex political encounter for radical and other feminists who see equality between the sexes as a core objective and patriarchy as the systematic oppression of women by men. For example, Christianity, Islam and Judaism are all highly patriarchal and it is only various forms of revisionism or reinterpretation that can assert otherwise. However, feminism is a common reference point for women of different faiths to frame their resistances within the religion and from external attacks on their choice to follow specific religious practices. This often relates to attacks on what is positioned as choice or free will to choose, for example, to pursue certain beliefs (Ghafournia, 2017) or to adhere to specific dress codes such as the hijab (Muslim women's headscarf). For example, a popular 'meme' on social media asserts "If woman is free to show her body why should she not be free to cover it?", accompanied by a picture of two young women dressed in hijabs, long sleeves, and long skirts.

For non-Muslim feminists seeking to work alongside self-defined Muslim feminists, it is important to be well informed about the struggles within communities rather than seeking to impose political strategies derived from their own contexts. Sarah Malik articulates a feminist Muslim position in the following:

> I'm at a wedding and my heart sinks. The Iman is smiling as he addresses a large South Asian banquet hall...The Iman proclaims how it is the duty of the groom to love and be kind to his wife, as if she were a dog or a child. He then reminds the bride to respect and obey the authority of her husband. This seems at best benign and paternalistic. But it is just one example of how male guardianship and authority proliferates in Muslim faith communities. It is a form of control that has a profound impact on women seeking divorce and religious mediation in marital disputes, and normalizes the social policing of women's movements, behavior and even dress, the kind of control that defines domestic violence. In part in is because of the problematic Quranic verse 4:34, which is misused by some men to claim superiority over women. It's an evasion to say beliefs in male headship are only cultural when the framework of guardianship asserted in understandings of this verse informs roles and expectations of women.
>
> *(Malik, 2017)*

Malik (2017) observed that the challenge for Muslim feminists is great, that they need to respond to the policing of women and the various forms of discrimination within Muslim communities and they must 'fight patriarchy in their communities'. Malik and other feminist Muslim writers assert that there have been strong feminist narratives in the tradition of Islam and much like other cultural struggles with dominant patriarchal structures, it has scapegoated feminism 'as antithetical to the culture and an alien Western affront and ignores the feminist narratives embedded in the tradition itself' (Malik, 2017).

Asserting a view from a Southeast Asian perspective, Aihwa Ong describes Western international feminism as 'strategic sisterhood' and suggests that it holds inherent disregard to other moral systems and ethics by proposing global human standards (2007, p. 31). Ong's (2007) response to global feminist strategies, such as 'women's rights are human rights', is drawn from a postcolonial nation perspective, where, in her view, there is a persistent threat of re-colonisation by constructing Southeast Asian women as in need of help and universalising their plight and needs for equality from an external Western point of view. Writing about social transformations in Malaysia, Ong sees a distinctive set of transformations taking place that are outside the Western feminist project. She observed that:

> Because postcolonial milieus are constantly unfolding, the question of women's emancipation is becoming less of a stark choice between universal feminist values or domestic political agendas. Instead of a dichotomy between feminist internationalism and female dominated nationalism, the postcolonial milieu in Southeast Asia is shaped by the intersection of nationalism, capitalist development, and religious institutions. The women-state patriarchal link is itself undergoing change, thus creating an opening for feminist claims against religious patriarchy.
>
> *(2007, pp. 32–33)*

Anti-imperialist feminist, Serene Khader (2018) argues that the single principle for transnational feminism must be based on ending sexist oppression and that this can be achieved by decolonising feminism from Western moral positions often presented as normative values within universal feminism. The values she points to that should be delinked from a shared feminist praxis with the global South, are aligned with populist or neoliberal feminisms' values. These include 'individualism, autonomy (and its associations with secular worldviews), and gender-role elimativism' (Khader, 2018, p. 3). Her view is based on a critique of disjuncture between global South values related to tradition, family, community, and religion with the white liberal/neoliberal values of global North feminists who see themselves as saviours of women in the global South. Khader is very strongly in favour of a transnational feminist praxis but seeks to orient the praxis from a global South point of view to avoid re-colonising tendencies of Western feminisms. She clearly states that 'feminism requires universalist opposition to sexist oppression, but feminism does not require universal adoption of Western "Enlightenment liberal" values and strategies' (2018, p. 4). Khader's argument includes an inherent critique of the dominance of neoliberal ideals that set out to determine 'which goods and power should be allocated' rather than the singular objective of ending sexist oppression, which 'mostly makes a point about how goods and power should be allocated' (2018, p. 4). In relation to social welfare (seen mostly in international development), Khader's (2018) position demands a clear-eyed view of the impact of uncritical assumptions about free-market capitalism benefiting women in the global South, which accompanies Western economic and social welfare interventions. The idea of Western progress as the ideal has largely not benefited women or local communities as the contemporary re-colonisation through economic development ends with resources accumulating with elites (often foreign corporations), as it did under colonisation.

Although it appears as, and often is, an attack on hegemonic Western feminisms, the diverse analyses of feminism from insider perspectives, in non-Western countries, further demonstrates the durability and irrepressibility of feminist practice. Just as it has been recognised through moments of historical resistance, feminist practice happens in all contexts, regardless of the odds against what Western feminism may see as standard gains for feminism. In Saudi Arabia, a country with obviously oppressive conditions and limited rights for women, the government announced a series of reforms in 2019, although many of the women who fought for reforms were on trial or in detention for their actions calling for women's rights (Human Rights Watch, 2019). The reforms included a decree allowing Saudi women to obtain a passport and travel abroad without approval from a male relative, as well register the birth of their child and were given some new protections against employment discrimination (Human Rights Watch, 2019). The significance of these and other reforms, including allowing Saudi women to drive a car, are the first challenges to the country's male guardianship system, a system that has allowed men to significantly 'control Saudi women's lives from birth until death' (Human Rights Watch, 2019). Human Rights Watch (2019) reported that as the new 'freedoms' were granted, the government cracked down on feminist activists, arresting many for acts of treason and subjecting them to imprisonment, torture, sexual harassment and assault. In 2021, the prominent Saudi women's rights activist, Loujain al-Hathloul was released from prison after being detained for 1,001 days, having been charged with pushing a foreign agenda (Chulov, 2021). Her release, however, was probationary and she was not allowed to travel or speak of her ordeal in prison (Chulov, 2021). Many other women remain imprisoned, as an apparent warning to others not to take public action for women's rights. Results from a study on recent advances in women's empowerment found that 'there is gender equality in education, but moderate results were perceived regarding gender equality in terms of job opportunities, financial returns, promotions and position' and the availability of non-feminised educational programmes and childcare (Alessa et al., 2022, p. 327). It appears that the wider environment for women's economic participation has improved in relation to education, leading to possible gains in women's social welfare, even though limitations on their rights to protest remain.

Despite such examples of resistance and a global reach within the women's movement, feminism as a social force for change has not been entirely successful from a global perspective. Gains for women's equality are patchy and proportionally marginal in many parts of the world. Despite the widespread number of women's non-governmental and institutional organisations established to achieve gender equality, there are still many women whom, because they are women, suffer extreme oppression, systematic and random violence (often sanctioned and ignored, if not protected by states) and second-class citizenship. The dominance of religious and ideological views that still privilege men's needs or value over women would suggest that feminism has failed to transform many traditional patriarchal structures in many societies across the global North as well as the global South (Phillips, 2015; Rosche, 2016; UNPD, 2015).

Women's/Feminist NGOs

In viewing feminism as a global movement and global practice, it is important to consider how it is sustained and perpetuated. It is evident that international institutions and states play a key role as well as feminist scholars and politicians, but it is through informal and formal non-governmental organisations (the third sector) that feminist practice has been and continues to be most strongly supported and sustained. In exploring theoretical explanations for the growth of interest and public visibility of feminism this book views the third sector (inclusive of all not-for-profit, civil society organisations) as a key component of a well-functioning pluralist democracy and a core vehicle for feminist practice in all political contexts, in terms of advocacy, service delivery and policy influence. Despite the proliferation of women's/feminist NGOs working for gender equality, in advocacy and the provision of services for women across the world, and after nearly 50 years of a worldwide feminist movement, there is no widespread recognition of basic feminist objectives as intrinsic to the functioning of a democracy. Indeed, many gains of the women's movement and third-sector feminist activists have faced significant backlashes and, in some cases, complete erosion in countries that are considered to be well-functioning democracies. Successive democratically elected conservative governments have routinely turned back the clock on hard fought for gains by women gained under more progressive governments. This became starkly obvious in the 2016 USA election of the Republican Party and its President Donald Trump who embraced a misogynistic, hyper-masculine characterisation in his campaign for president and once elected set about reversing key legislative gains such as reproductive and health rights for women both in the USA and internationally through restrictions on aid (Girard, 2017). Not only did Trump defeat the first woman to run for president likely to win, but his agenda also prompted fear and grief:

> The nearly two-year-long election season that led to the surprising announcement early on Wednesday morning has been one of the most volatile, controversial and bitterly contested ever to take place, with many women now left mourning over the loss of a potential landmark in feminism and fearing what a Trump presidency means for them…Reactions of grief poured in on social media: "What's even more demoralising is knowing how hard Hillary's worked and how qualified she is, and yet… And every woman knows this feeling," said writer and columnist Anne Donahue on <u>Twitter</u>. In a similar sentiment, feminist writer Jessica Valenti <u>tweeted</u> that this is "what backlash looks like - to women's rights, to racial progress, to a cultural shift that doesn't centre white men."
>
> *(Sarhan, 2016)*

Reflecting extreme right and Christian fundamentalist, anti-choice values Trump asserted that women should be punished for having abortions and his appointment of anti-abortion judges to the Supreme Court reflected a simmering resentment of the groups with which he aligned himself, along with Vice President Pence and his team of Presidential advisors, all of whom present as anti-feminist and against the rights of lesbian, gay, bisexual, trans and queer (LGBTQ) peoples (Girard, 2017, p. 1). Trump's presidency has been characterised by the maintenance of white male power both symbolically, legislatively and regarding his appointments into key positions of leadership, making his reign emblematic of conservative governments' backlash against feminism's gains.

Although Raewyn Connell (2019) has described the influence of women's and feminist ally men's NGOs as a light touch in terms of global politics, 'no more than a cry in the wind', in the face of authoritarian male leaders, I argue that they have been critical in terms of women's participation in policy development and social welfare outcomes for women, and continue to be a form of resistance in the face of global shifts towards anti-feminist and misogynist politics. As Connell notes, however:

> There are doubtless thousands of NGOs working on gender issues, if you add them up: in research, health services, lobbying, media, counselling, public advocacy, education and more. The international network of pro-feminist men's groups, MenEngage Alliance (www.menengage.org), which works on violence prevention and changing attitudes among men, claims six or seven hundred affiliates. There is impressive creativity in the NGO terrain. One cannot say, however, that this form of activism has generated a particular kind of theory, in the way women's liberation generated radical feminism and socialist feminism, and a later generation produced queer theory and trans feminism. Most NGOs I know of, and most contemporary public-sector agencies concerned with gender issues, seem to work comfortably with a loose liberal feminism. That is to say, they presume a simple dichotomy between women and men; they celebrate the advancement of individual women into management and political office; their rhetoric centres on the idea of equal rights; they hope for, and sometimes work for, a change in men's attitudes. 'Women's rights are human rights' is a familiar principle — as if human rights were unassailable. These ideas have practical value. They justify funding for women's health services, equal educational provision for girls, anti-discrimination measures and campaigns against domestic violence. But they do not address gross economic disparities, and they do not give much grip on the new power structures of transnational corporate management.
>
> *(2019, p. 60)*

To advance Connell's (2019) idea of practical value, feminist practice has succeeded in influencing global social policies in the case of the United Nations' Sustainable Development Goals (UN SDGs), where it is clearly evident that substantial feminist ideas and critique have brought about a reframing of the UN

Millennium Development Goals (UN MDGs) due to their widespread failure to reach goals that were set to achieve genuine gender equality targets (Phillips, 2015; Rosche, 2016). One of the outstanding aspects of the development of the UN MDGs and the UN SDGs was the participation and influence of NGOs, as noted below by Daniela Rosche, a feminist working in the international NGO sector:

> The formulation of the Agenda 2030 and the Sustainable Development Goals (SDGs) have involved greater consultation with civil society than their predecessors, the Millennium Development Goals. This has been welcome to many development non-government organisations undertaking advocacy on women's rights and gender equality, which have engaged with the SDG process in various ways.
>
> *(Rosche, 2016, p. 111)*

Rosche (2016) documented the process by which Oxfam (Netherlands) and its global network of Oxfam branches, developed its own focus on women and gender equality and embarked on a radical advocacy agenda to influence the new UN SDGs after recognising the limitations and failures in relation to gender equality of the UN MDGs. Pinpointing the lack of a rights-based approach and thus failing to 'lay the necessary groundwork to bring about the transformational change needed to give women greater control over their own lives' as a key failure in the MDGs, and it was seen as 'ineffective in addressing the systemic manifestations of women's subordination such as intimate partner violence and the unpaid care burden' Oxfam developed a 'women's rights influencing strategy' (Rosche, 2016, pp. 113–114). Their strategy included the objective of reaching a consensus that there should be a specific gender goal for the 2015 to 2030 UN SDG plan, consensus amongst the stakeholders was achieved and Oxfam's core foci on policy development related to violence against women and the 'unpaid care burden' were eventually successfully incorporated into Goal 5 of the UN SDGs. This was achieved through persistent feminist practice conducted via a network of feminist practitioners within the NGO sector:

> One of the earliest calls for such a stand-alone gender goal coming from feminists within the development NGOs sector was made in a joint alliance paper published in January 2013 by the UK's GADN (2013). The paper succeeds in making a compelling case, based on strong gender analysis of poverty, why a stand-alone gender goal in the new post-2105 was needed.
>
> *(Rosche, 2016, p. 115)*

The final Goal 5 of the UN SDGs included the agenda collectively developed by Oxfam and other NGO feminists. It became a strong formulation for improving women's social welfare across the world and aiming to address the gross economic disparities experienced by many of the world's women because they are women. It included targets to:

- End all forms of discrimination against all women and girls everywhere
- Eliminate all forms of violence against all women and girls in the public and private spheres, including trafficking and sexual and other types of exploitation
- Eliminate all harmful practices, such as child, early and forced marriage and female genital mutilation
- Recognise and value unpaid care and domestic work through the provision of public services, infrastructure and social protection policies and the promotion of shared responsibility within the household and the family as nationally appropriate
- Ensure women's full and effective participation and equal opportunities for leadership at all levels of decision-making in political, economic and public life
- Ensure universal access to sexual and reproductive health and reproductive rights as agreed in accordance with the Programme of Action of the International Conference on Population and Development and the Beijing Platform for Action and the outcome documents of their review conferences
- Undertake reforms to give women equal rights to economic resources, as well as access to ownership and control over land and other forms of property, financial services, inheritance and natural resources, in accordance with national laws
- Enhance the use of enabling technology, in particular information and communications technology, to promote the empowerment of women
- Adopt and strengthen sound policies and enforceable legislation for the promotion of gender equality and the empowerment of all women and girls at all levels (UNSDGs, 2016).

The SDG 5 agenda represents the aspirations of organised women's NGOs and their knowledge derived from relations with grassroots level needs of women. It also reflects the slow and ineffectual progress of prior global policy commitments for women's equality. In setting this agenda, the collaborative efforts of NGOs, governments and international institutions have captured the global state of social welfare for women, offering a blueprint for policy for change, but also a very clear picture of gender inequality.

To a large extent, scholarly analysis of feminist praxis such as the SDG 5 objectives leads to an impasse between feminist revisionism related to 'gender' and the anti-structuralism that was linked to it. The recent rise in popularity of postcolonial, intersectional and standpoint feminisms in academic research and wide feminist practice have contributed to feminist paths that embrace a hybridity in approaches to the tensions between individualist gender approaches and the feminist collectivism that seems to be necessary for social change. This type of feminist praxis signals a resistance to and direct critique of the influence of neoliberalism and its influence on international development and aid programs, particularly in relation to the nature of individualised empowerment strategies (Phillips, 2015). It also reinforces a view of postfeminism as an exclusively white, global North concept of women's contemporary status where, as Rosalind Gill noted 'it present[s] women as autonomous agents no longer constrained by any inequalities in power imbalances whatsoever' (2007, p. 153).

Despite the promotion of the idea of postfeminism in countries such as Australia, the UK and the USA, feminism as both an identity and as a practice is alive and well and has re-emerged in those countries with an increased, often debated public presence over the last half-decade or so. Postfeminism has been utilised as a neat neoliberal, anti-feminist construct that has been promoted by decision-makers who are blind to inequality and deny their own sexism or even misogyny. From a global perspective, feminisms thrive as resistance and critique as well as an increasingly recognised framework for social justice and social transformation. Within both Southern and Northern scholarship, there has been extensive theorisation about the nature and extent of feminism and its role in social transformation on a global scale. Much feminist scholarship is critical and self-reflexive and constantly challenges generalisations about what feminism is, how it can be applied and for whom it exists. However, feminist theory and scholarship, by its very nature, have always allowed for self-defined feminist identity, and social and geographical diversity in how that identity is asserted and understood.

One of the most forceful critiques of the relationship between feminism and feminist practice within women's NGOs, is the 'NGOisation paradigm' (Hodžić, 2014, p. 221). Hodžić describes this as the organisation of feminist knowledge about NGOs by feminist scholars that by its narrow perspectives of the formation of women's and feminist NGOs' effects on the women's movement, 'constrains the space of analysis and critique' (2014, p. 222). The NGOisation critique was a response to the rapid rise and growth of feminist and women's NGOs during the 1990s. As an anti-institutional response, it positioned NGOs as harmful to feminism and as a distraction from and corruption of the goals of the women's movement through alignment with the state, bureaucratisation of women's organising and exploitation of women's labour (Hodžić, 2014, pp. 222–223). With plenty of evidence of the failure of NGOs to deliver more broadly, this view is part of a wider critique of NGOs that have become large and highly bureaucratic, operating from the global North but delivering services and assistance in the global South. A critical perspective of NGOisation sees it as a form of neo-colonialist intervention into the lives of usually former colonies of the Northern NGO's home country that effectively dampens the capacity for local political action and collectivist responses to social, economic, and sometimes cultural problems. At the very least, this critique demands a critical perspective on the long-term impact of an NGO at the grassroots level. For example, are the actions of the NGO enough to challenge deeply entrenched oppressions such as gender inequality? Do they open spaces for local women to speak and be listened to and have input into their own welfare and economic or social transformations? These are important questions for feminists working in the international context of providing or advocating for social welfare in general but particularly pertinent for feminist praxis. The postcolonial feminist demand for grassroots women's voices to be heard (Mohanty, 2003; Spivak, 2010) and contribute to decisions about social assistance and social protection is a crucial global South position for feminist praxis within international NGOs.

Global Inequality

The pay gap between men and women is a persistent problem confronted by feminists for many decades now. Inequality of income is closely linked to the feminisation of poverty and international comparisons tend to reflect overall gender inequalities. In their 2021 Global Gender Gap report, the World Economic Forum (WEF) reported that even in the best-performing country, Sweden, there is still an 18 per cent income gap between men and women. In other global North countries, there is also a persistent gap of, for example, 38 per cent in Denmark, 39 per cent in France and 35 per cent in the USA. In many countries in the global South, the gap is extreme, for example, Yemen had the largest income gap, where women's income is only 7 per cent of men's income, creating an income gap of over 93 per cent (WEF, 2021). These data show that even in the most advanced 'gender equal' societies there are still stark differences in women's wage and economic equality, roles in governance in both public and private spheres, some occupational and academic fields and representation in politics. Research also shows that women suffer greater poverty than men and due to the failure in addressing specific health needs such as maternal health and equal rights in relation to marriage, are at greater risk of mortality from treatable medical conditions or interpersonal violence (Hughes et al., 2015; UN Women, 2015, p. 3).

What is evident when data on women's global inequality are examined is that women suffer the most disadvantage in countries that, along with poor access to education, unequal pay, and low political participation, have weak social welfare provision and poor labour regulation. Although varying in degrees, and not the only source of welfare in most societies, a strong welfare state is evidence of economic stability and democratic governance and mostly where a strong women's voice has been heard in social policy development. However, in more complex social and economic environments there is wide variation in how different women experience social welfare and gender equality policies. For example, in an in-depth analysis of the economic impact of the global COVID-19 pandemic the WEF found evidence that although everyone was severely affected, it was women who experienced more significant effects through 'multiple channels' (WEF, 2021, p. 43). The impact of the pandemic on women related to their more common employment in sectors most directly disrupted by lockdowns and by social distancing measures and women's re-employment, which was more subdued than men, resulting in a lowering of workforce participation. The analysis also indicated 'lower hiring rates and delayed hiring into leadership roles', and more reduced hours than men upon returning to work, as well as greater job losses for women world-wide (5 per cent as compared to 3.9 per cent for men) (WEF, 2021, pp. 43–44). A further finding related to 'a more severe "doubleshift"'(WEF, 2021, p. 43). Although a common experience for women with caring responsibilities, there was clearly an increase in the 'overlap of work responsibilities and care (house-work, childcare and eldercare) responsibilities' (WEF, 2021, p. 43). Although there was evidence of men becoming more involved in unpaid work at home, it was not surprising that most caring and home management responsibilities fell dispropor-tionally on women. Measures such as school closures and isolation of informal car-ers, causing changes to care arrangements, were key aspects of 'widening labour force participation gender gaps', reemphasising how childcare is an enabler for women's labour force participation (WEF, 2021, p. 43). Another, more invisible impact on women's welfare, in the Australian context at least, related to a govern-ment pandemic policy that allowed people to withdraw funds prematurely from their retirement savings (superannuation) if they had lost income due to the pan-demic. According to The Australian Institute of Superannuation Trustees, more than 70,000 women appeared to have experienced coercive financial abuse since the release scheme began early in 2020, instances where abusive husbands forced their spouses to withdraw money from their future retirement savings (Curtis, 2022). This meant for some women they were now destined to suffer a similar experience of potential poverty to their mothers or grandmothers, whom in their thirties and forties had no savings for their retirement due to exclusion from the paid workforce as home-based carers earlier in their adult lives (Curtis, 2022).

Another example of economic burden for women during crises was during the financial crisis in Europe beginning in 2007 and 2008, which imposed a sustained era of austerity, and gender equality policies were demoted by the European Union (EU) (Cullen, 2015). The impact of marginalising gender equality policy and activities by the EU resulted in 'a mixture of long-term shifts away from binding legislation on equal treatment to soft law initiatives around gender mainstreaming, diversity, and equality mainstreaming' (Cullen, 2015, p. 411). The prior focus on gender-equality programmes within the EU is attributable to the work of feminist NGOs, in particular the European Wom-en's Lobby (EWL), which represented 4,000 other women's organisations, and their capacity to engage institutionally with the governance structure of the EU (Cullen, 2015). Further, UN Women's (2014) analysis of the impact of the Global Financial Crisis in Europe and the USA demonstrated that despite the overall welfare or level of economic advancement of a country, women suffered greater poverty than men in an economic downturn because of their existing levels of feminised poverty and social exclusion. UN Women reported that in 2011 there were 8 million more women at risk of poverty than men across the EU countries and in six of the 31 EU countries the ratio of women's risk of poverty over men was 120 (UN Women 2014). Although the outlook could be far worse, global estimates for 2022 were that 388 million women and girls would be experiencing extreme poverty, in comparison to an estimated 372 million men and boys (UN Women, 2022). This estimated level of poverty for women and girls has been greatly affected by the impact of the Coronavirus pandemic. However, according to UN Women (2022), projected poverty levels could be addressed by increasing spending on social protection (social welfare), investing in a sustainable green economy, improving infrastructure and education, and claim it would lift around 150 million women and girls out of poverty by 2030.

A gendered risk of poverty is far greater for women aged over 65, whose material deprivation rate in 2012 was 8.6 per cent compared to 6.1 per cent for men in the same age group (UN Women, 2014). It is this connection in the wider sphere of material deprivation for older women that offers a unique positionality for this book. Due to the intrinsic task of motherhood and the traditional, gendered roles of the primary carer parent, women are both the key users of welfare services as well as the key deliverers of welfare in all communities. A discussion of welfare without a focus on women is more than a half-empty discussion and there has been a growing awareness of this over the past 20 years or so, hence the emphasis on gender in development and the recognition of women in key role in the business of families.

From a global perspective, women's social welfare is firmly on the agenda of international institutions and global social policy agendas, as encapsulated by the orientation of several of the UN SDG goals and the now consistent, annual research into gender inequality by powerful institutions such as the WEF and the OECD. The fundamental recognition of poverty as the greatest threat to welfare and well-being and that, on a global and national scale, women are at greater risk of poverty than their male counterparts, has been a key driver for institutions and states to act or at least respond with gender equality policies and assistance programs. Solving high global levels of gendered inequality in welfare or social protection is highly challenging and states' official donor aid and UN programs can only operate successfully through strong partnerships with receiver countries and the many NGOs that are now likely deliverers of social welfare in states with weak or no welfare states. As discussed above, feminist praxis strongly resides within women's NGOs across the world (Phillips, 2015) but state engagement with how women are targeted and assisted is not necessarily informed by feminism or understandings of women's rights and gender inequality. Also, due to the ever-changing politics of some governments, the progress of such initiatives is unpredictable, reversible and often immeasurable. Sweden is the only government to have established an explicitly feminist foreign policy (in 2014), which aimed to enhance Sweden's gender equality focus through its engagement in international security, trade, and development. The Swedish policy was built on a commitment to gender equality as a precursor for strong economic development and the inclusion of women's voices in peace and security (Government Offices of Sweden, 2021).

In contrast, in the contemporary global context, the political re-emergence of populism and authoritarianism has brought with it a renewed wave of anti-feminism, homophobia and misogyny, a backlash far greater than what confronted feminists in the global North in the 1990s. As Raewyn Connell notes:

> Political power in many parts of the world has been grasped by groups of men — there are no women in this list — who operate a strategy of authoritarian populism. Of course, there are large differences among them; but also important similarities, including their gender politics. Most mobilize racism and nationalism, most have cashed in on border protection and fear of terrorism, most are anti-feminist, homophobic and celebrate strong conventional masculinity.
>
> *(2019, p. 60)*

This trend was evident in global North countries such as Hungary, Poland, and the USA under Trump where women have lost rights such as reproductive choice and have been exposed to direct sexism from leaders. Similar sexist attacks on women and women's rights have also occurred in the global South, in Brazil, the Philippines and India for example. Although the WEF has ranked the Philippines highly regarding economic gender equality, President Duterte's rule has meant an extreme rise in sexism and violence against women. Time reported on protests against the Philippine president:

> Among those anti-government protesters are women's rights activists, who have increasingly been speaking out against the Duterte administration. Since taking office in June 2016, the 73-year-old leader has ordered soldiers to shoot female rebels "in the vagina," made inappropriate comments about his female Vice President's legs, joked about raping Miss Universe, and equated having a second wife to keeping a "spare tire" in the trunk of a car.
>
> *(Haynes, 2018)*

When a government leader models such attitudes towards women, control of and abuse and violence against women increases. Women's social welfare, along with other people targeted by right-wing populist hate such as people with diverse sexual identities and immigrant groups, is diminished. Feminist resistance, a key form of feminist practice, to such forces is crucial and plays a central role in social welfare for women and others victimised under this kind of rule. As will be noted throughout this book, feminist activism that has achieved major reforms in the past is being repeated as anti-feminist, populist conservatives gain power and laws and services that protect women's autonomy and welfare are withdrawn.

Conclusion

The aim of this chapter was to establish the global nature of the book via insights into the scope of feminism's influence in opposing sexism in all its forms and calling for gender equality in the global context. By presenting some differing global South perspectives on feminism and their relationships to global North feminism, the chapter opens the terrain of collaborative knowledge building and feminist critique. This establishes a connection with the positioning of different national and cultural experiences of feminism. This chapter has also explored the central organisational means for global feminist action and influence in a discussion of the role of NGOs and how they have acted as vehicles for global social policy influence, particularly in relation to the UN SDGs. The final section of the chapter illuminated global perspectives and data on gender inequality and international institutional interests in and recognition of the importance of gender inequality as a measure of the success of human and economic development. A key aspect of addressing global poverty rates is now based on well-researched understandings of women's disadvantage within and across national contexts. The most powerful international economic institutions are significantly investing in understanding the extent and impact of gender inequality in all countries in the world. Throughout the chapter, and continued as a theme in the following chapters, is an underlying critical reflection of the dominance of neoliberalism in global and national governance and economies, as well as how it has influenced and used feminism in its market orientation.

The broad themes explored in this chapter establish a background for the following chapters that focus on key areas of social welfare and feminist practice. As it was always the intention for this book to draw on the actions and experiences of feminist practitioners, the scope of the lived experiences of feminist action and struggle described in each chapter draws on a wide range of sources, mainstream media reports, scholarly research and alternative online accounts. The greatest challenge to pulling together a fair account of feminist practice and action was the everchanging nature of feminist achievements in everchanging social, political and environmental contexts. This means of course that there is nothing exhaustive about this book as it can only present mere moments in the expansive feminist project of social change on a global scale.

References

Abdel-Magied, Y. (2017) *Yassmin's Story*. North Sydney: Vintage Australia.

Alessa, N., Shalhoob, H.S. and Almugarry, H.A. (2022) Saudi women's economic empowerment in light of Saudi Vision 2030: Perception, challenges and opportunities. *Journal of Educational and Social Research*, 12 (1), 316–334.

Barry, K. (1979) *Female Sexual Slavery*. Englewood Cliffs, NJ: Prentice Hall.

Barry, K. (1995) *The Prostitution of Sexuality*. New York: New York University Press.

Baumgardner, J. (2011) Is there a fourth wave? Does it matter? From the book *F'em Goo Goo, Gaga and Some Thoughts on Balls*. https://www.feminist.com/resources/artspeech/genwom/baumgardner2011.html.

Bell, E., Meriläinen, S., Taylor, S. and Tienari, J. (2019) Time's up! Feminist theory and activism meets organization studies. *Human Relations*, 72 (1), 4–22.

Bowden, P. and Mummery, J. (2009) *Understanding Feminism*. Stocksfield: Acumen.

Carland, S. (2017) *Fighting Hislam, Women, Faith and Sexism.* Melbourne: Melbourne University Press.

Chulov, M. (2021) Saudi women's rights activist Loujain al-Hathloul released from prison. *The Guardian,* Thursday, February 11. https://www.theguardian.com/world/2021/feb/10/saudi-womens-rights-activist-loujain-al-hathloul-released-from-prison.

Connell, R. (2015) Meeting at the edge of fear: Theory on a world scale. *Feminist Theory,* 16 (1), 49–66.

Connell, R. (2019) New maps of struggle for gender justice: Rethinking feminist research on organizations and work. *Gender, Work, and Organization,* 26 (1), 54–63.

Cullen, P. (2015) Feminist NGOs and the European Union. Contracting opportunities and strategic response. *Social Movement Studies,* 14 (4), 410–426.

Curtis, K. (2022) 'A perfect storm': Up to 70,000 women may have been coerced into withdrawing super. *The Sydney Morning Herald,* February 21. https://www.smh.com.au/politics/federal/a-perfect-storm-up-to70-000-women-may-have-been-coerced-into-withdrawing-super-20220217-p59xac.html

David, M. (2014) *Feminism, Gender, and Universities: Politics, Passion, and Pedagogies.* Surrey; Burlington: Ashgate.

Dillon, Joanne (2007) Thirty years of feminist activism: Women in welfare education reflect. PhD thesis, Victoria University. https://vuir.vu.edu.au/30246/.

Dworkin, A. (1987) Pornography is civil rights issue for women. *University of Michigan Journal of Law Reform,* 21 (2), 55–68.

Dworkin, A. (1993) Prostitution and male supremacy. *Michigan Journal of Gender & Law,* 1 (1) 1–12.

Eschle, C. and Maiguashca, B. (2014) Reclaiming feminist futures: Co-opted and progressive politics in a neo-liberal age. *Political Studies,* 62 (3), 634–651.

Eyadat, Z. (2013) Islamic feminism: Roots, development and policies. *Global Policy,* 4 (4), 359–368.

Ghafournia, F. (2017) Muslim women and domestic violence: Developing a framework for social work practice. *Journal of Religion & Spirituality in Social Work,* 36 (1–2), 146–163.

Gill, R. (2007) Postfeminist media culture: Elements of a sensibility. *European Journal of Cultural Studies,* 10 (2), 147–166.

Gillis, S., Howie, G. and Munford, R. (2007) *Third Wave Feminism: A Critical Exploration.* Basingstoke: Palgrave Macmillan.

Girard, F. (2017) Implications of the Trump administration for sexual and reproductive rights globally. *Reproductive Health Matters,* 25 (49), 6–13.

Government Offices of Sweden (2021) *Gender Equality in Sweden: Feminist Government.* https://www.goverment.se/4a7738/contentassets/efcc5a15ef4522a872de46ad69148/gender-equality-policy-in-sweden

Gray, M. and Boddy, J. (2010) Making sense of the waves: Wipeout or still riding high? *Affilia: Journal of Women and Social Work,* 25 (4) 368–389.

Haynes, S. (2018) Women in the Philippines have had enough of President Duterte's 'Macho' Leadership'. *Time,* July 23, 2018. https://time.com/5345552/duterte-philippines-sexism-sona-women/.

Hodžić, S. (2014) Feminist bastards: Toward a posthumanist critique of NGOization. In V. Bernal and I. Grewal (eds) *Theorizing NGOs, States, Feminism and Neo-liberalism.* Durham; London: Duke University Press, 221–247.

Huffington Post (2016) French Law bans buying prostitutes, offering help instead of punishment, April 7. http://www.huffingtonpost.com/entry/french-law-bans-buying-sex-but-protects-prostitutes_us_57052fd7e4b0b90ac270d6f6.

Hughes, C., Bolis, M., Fries, R. and Finigan, S. (2015) Women's economic inequality and domestic violence: Exploring the links and empowering women. *Gender & Development*, 23 (2), 279–297.

Human Rights Watch (2019) Saudi Arabia: Important advances for Saudi women freedom to obtain passports, but women activists remained jailed. *Human Rights Watch Website*. https://www.hrw.org/news/2019/08/02/saudi-arabia-important-advances-saudi-women.

Khader, S.J. (2018) *Decolonizing Universalism: A Transnational Feminist Ethic*. New York: Oxford University Press.

Leupold, L. (2010) *Fourth Way Feminism*, Special Report. Portfolio Magazine. http://journalism.nyu.edu/publishing/archives/portfolio/leupold/.

MacKinnon, C.A. (1985) Pornography, civil rights, and speech. *Harvard Civil Rights-Civil Liberties. Law Review*, 20, 1–70.

Malik, S. (2017) How can Muslim feminists reclaim their religion from men? *ABC News*, May 1. http://www.abc.net.au/news/2017-05-01/how-muslim-feminists-can-reclaim-religion-men/8484994.

Marcos, S. and Waller, M. (2016) *Dialogue and Difference: Feminisms Challenge Globalization*. New York and Houndmills: Palgrave Macmillan.

Marks, E. and De Courtivron, I. (1980) *New French Feminisms: An Anthology*. Amherst: University of Massachusetts Press.

McRobbie, A. (ed.) (2009) *The Aftermath of Feminism*. Los Angeles and London: SAGE Publications.

McRobbie, A. (2015) Notes on the perfect: Competitive femininity in neoliberal times. *Australian Feminist Studies*, 30 (83), 3–20.

Mohanty, C.T. (2003) *Feminism without Borders Decolonizing Theory, Practicing Solidarity*. Durham: Duke University Press.

Murphy, M. (2016) Women won't be silenced at Australia's first abolitionist conference. *Feminist Current*, April 8. http://www.feministcurrent.com/2016/04/08/women-wont-be-silenced-at-australias-first-abolitionist-conference/.

OECD (2020) *Gender Equality*. OECD Gender Initiative. https://www.oecd.org/gender/.

Ong, A. (2007) *Neoliberalism as Exception: Mutations of Citizenship and Sovereignty*. Durham: Duke University Press.

Phillips, R. (2015) How 'empowerment' may miss its mark: Gender equality policies and how they are understood in women's NGOs. *Voluntas: International Journal of Voluntary and Nonprofit Organizations*, 26 (4), 1122–1142.

Phillips, R. and Cree, V.E. (2014) What does the 'fourth wave' mean for teaching feminism in twenty-first century social work? *Social Work Education: The International Journal*, 33 (7), 930–943.

Phipps, A. (2020) *Me, Not You: The Trouble with Mainstream Feminism*. Manchester: Manchester University Press.

Rosche, D. (2016) Agenda 2030 and the sustainable development goals: Gender equality at last? An Oxfam perspective. *Gender & Development*, 24 (1), 111–126.

Rottenberg, C. (2014) The rise of neoliberal feminism. *Cultural Studies*, 28 (3), 418–437.

Sarhan, J. (2016) What a Donald Trump victory means for women. *Aljazeera News*, November 10. https://www.aljazeera.com/features/2016/11/10/what-a-donald-trump-victory-means-for-women.

Shaw, C.M. (2015) *Women and Power in Zimbabwe, Promises of Feminism*. Champaign: University of Illinois Press.

Simões, R.B., Amaral, I. and José, S.S. (2021) The new feminist frontier on community-based learning. Popular feminism, online misogyny, and toxic masculinities. *European Journal for Research on the Education and Learning of Adults*, 12 (2), 165–177.

Spivak, G.C. (2010) Can the subaltern speak? In R.C. Morris (ed.) Revised Edition, from the 'History' Chapter of Critique of Postcolonial Reason. *Can the Subaltern Speak?: Reflections on the History of an Idea.* New York: Columbia University Press, 21–78.

UNDP (United Nations Development Program) (2015) *Human Development Report.* Chapter 4, Imbalances in Paid and Unpaid Work, 107–137. https://hdr.undp.org/sites/default/files/2015_human_development_report_0.pdf.

UNMDGs (2013) *The Millennium Development Goals Report.* New York: United Nations. https://www.un.org/millenniumgoals/pdf/report-2013/mdg-report-2013-english.pdf.

UNSDGs (2016) *Sustainable Development Goals.* Geneva: United Nations. (Accessed May 23, 2017). http://www.un.org/sustainabledevelopment/sustainable-development-goals/.

UNSDGs (2022) *The SDGs in Action.* UNPD. https://www.undp.org/sustainable-development-goals.

UN Women (2014) *The Global Economic Crisis and Gender Equality.* New York: UN Women. https://www.unwomen.org/sites/default/files/Headquarters/Attachments/Sections/Library/Publications/2014/TheGlobalEconomicCrisisAndGenderEquality-en%20pdf.pdf.

UN Women (2015) *The Global Economic Crisis and Gender Equality.* New York: UN Women. http://www.unwomen.org/~/media/headquarters/attachments/sections/library/publications/2014/theglobaleconomiccrisisandgenderequality-en%20pdf.ashx.

UN Women (2022) *Poverty Deepens for Women and Girls, According to Latest Projections.* New York: Un Women. https://data.unwomen.org/features/poverty-deepens-women-and-girls-according-latest-projections.

Walby, S. (2011) The impact of feminism on sociology. *Sociological Research Online,* 16 (3), 1–10.

WHO (World Health Organisation) (2021) *The Future We Expect: Women's Health and Gender Equality.* World Health Organisation. https://www.who.int/news/item/28-06-2021-the-future-we-expect-women-s-health-and-gender-equality.

World Economic Forum (WEF) (2021) Global gender report 2021. *Insight Report March 2021.* https://www3.weforum.org/docs/WEF_GGGR_2021.pdf.

3

DOMESTIC VIOLENCE

Feminism and Feminist Practice

Introduction

First, this chapter will discuss how the extent and impact of domestic violence creates extensive needs for social welfare and how it is presented and responded to as a 'problem' in social policy. Second, it focuses on feminism's significant contribution to theory, policy and practice as they relate to domestic violence. Finally, it asks key questions. Why is there still extensive, worldwide violence against women? Is a fresh analysis of power and domination required for effective feminist social welfare practice? How can new perspectives be negotiated within a contemporary feminist context? Also, can feminist welfare practitioners work to shape criminal justice and wider social response to domestic violence?

From the outset, it is important to recognise that the term 'domestic violence' is often used interchangeably with terms such as 'violence against women', 'domestic abuse', 'family violence', 'intimate partner violence', 'interpersonal violence' and others. In some cases, there are distinctions made between these terms based on gender (in same-sex relationships for example) and other family member inclusion. USA-based research has shown that in lesbian, gay, bisexual, queer, intersex and asexual (GLBTQIA+) communities there are higher rates of domestic violence compared with heterosexual and cisgender communities (Costello and Greenwald, 2022). It is further recognised that people of colour, immigrants and/or disabled people within such communities are at the highest risk of domestic violence, linked to discrimination and violence in the wider, heteronormative community (Costello and Greenwald, 2022) thus demonstrating intersectional complexities minority gender groups face.

However, in general, most research and terms related to domestic violence relate to violence committed against cis-gender women, including women in same-sex relationships. The cisgender focus is due to the predominance of

DOI: 10.4324/9781315625188-3

normative heterosexual relationships across the world and the overwhelming research and evidence that demonstrates women are most commonly victims of domestic violence. It is recognised that children within relationships where there is domestic violence are also deeply affected and suffer many of the adverse consequences of the violence and substantial research conducted across the world shows that pregnant women experience extreme vulnerabilities to violence from an intimate partner (Garg et al., 2019; Naghizadeh et al., 2021; Orpin et al., 2020). Many studies of incidence and harm are conducted by medical researchers but the interest in conducting such research has arisen from pressure by feminists to address the high-level incidence of domestic violence. Feminist practitioners and researchers have also been successful in deepening an understanding of the forms that domestic violence takes, pushing the limited, early understanding from physical abuse to include, sexual abuse, marital rape, emotional abuse, psychological abuse, financial abuse and coercive control. The World Health Organisation estimates that, worldwide, 27 per cent of women between the ages of 15 years to 49 years have experienced domestic violence (WHO, 2021). Although not a focus in this chapter, violence against women can occur on institutional and societal levels through religious, cultural and legal mechanisms that mean women and other minority genders are harmed because of their gender. Such harms have naturally been a concern of feminisms' broad resistance and motivation to push for global gender equality and are alluded to in other sections of this book.

A large proportion of social welfare practice in response to domestic violence, in the provision of safety, prevention, behaviour change and legal services or interventions, will involve the safety of children. There is also an important feminist argument that 'violence against women' should include all forms of violence, including sexual assault, sexual harassment, online trolling, systemic, patriarchal impositions such as female genital mutilation, honour killings, forced marriage, child brides and acid attacks (Hester, 2004). I agree that there are many parallels in the reasons why all forms of violence against women, including transwomen, are connected to gender/power relationships and that this approach should be incorporated into broad policy objectives, conventions and legislation (McQuigg, 2018). Acknowledged in this chapter as a crucial feminist perspective, some examples of wider, systemic forms of violence against women are included, where feminists have been able to make inroads and resistances to those forms of violence. The specific field of domestic violence is a very significant area of feminist social welfare practice, especially in the practice and research of social work (Orme, 2003). Therefore, this chapter will mostly focus on intimate partner violence against women as domestic violence (and the consequential impact on their children). First, it is important to assess the broader societal problem of violence against women. In doing so, domestic violence and violence against women will be the favoured, interchangeable terms as they have important aetiologies linked to feminism, which will be elaborated on later in this chapter.

Feminist Practice against Domestic Violence

It is fair to say that there is no other area of practice in social welfare, health or social work that has been more influenced or framed by feminism than domestic violence. Overwhelming evidence and documented experiences of domestic violence do, and always have revealed the predominance of violence of men against women. Historically, the deep and abiding gendered nature of interpersonal violence between women and men who are intimate partners, was for so long hidden in the folds of the private domestic sphere and it was feminist activists, often women who had endured or witnessed violence in their own families, who dragged it into the public sphere for it to be recognised as both a societal and a social policy problem. Prior to the successful voicing of domestic violence as a common experience, facilitated by both the literal collective empowerment of women to speak of their own experiences through feminist political action and feminist theorisation to understand it, it was not regarded a social policy issue. As a widespread social phenomenon, across all cultures, domestic violence was a silent problem, known of but allowed to remain in the domain of the rights of men to act out their personal power against the women in their lives.

Nancy Fraser (2013) effectively summarised how feminists asserted domestic violence onto the political agenda in the USA:

> Until the 1970s, the expression "wife battering" did not exist. When spoken of publicly at all, this phenomenon was called "wife-beating" and was often treated comically, as in "have you stopped beating your wife?" Classed linguistically with the disciplining of children and servants, it was cast as "domestic", as opposed to a "political" matter. Then feminists renamed the practice with a term drawn from criminal law and created a new kind of public discourse. They claimed that battery was not a personal, domestic problem but a systemic political one; its aetiology was not to be traced to individual women's or men's emotional problems but, rather, to the ways these problems refracted pervasive social relations of male dominance and female subordination.
>
> *(Fraser, 2013, p. 72)*

However, as Fraser (2013) further elaborates, the success of making wife-battery or domestic violence a political issue and the achievement of forcing it onto the social policy agenda of governments, resulting in agreement to provide state or government support for shelters and other services, resulted in challenges to feminist principles and practice. As in other countries where the women's movement made similar gains in the 1970s, the initial means of addressing the needs of women affected by interpersonal violence were addressed by collectives of women who had shared the experiences or were political activists acting in solidarity with women who needed shelter or refuge to escape violence (Bowstead, 2015; Hester, 2004; Murray and Powell, 2009). The services were non-hierarchical and often saw the women who used the services as potential feminist activists.

However, once they were government funded and regulated, the refuges became subject to administrative demands, professionalisation and instrumentalisation (for the state). This saw the shift of refuges or shelters into a form of welfare rather than a form of resistance against men's violence and, as Fraser (2013) points out, shelters became more individualising and politicised. By professionalising the services for women escaping violence, the women were then positioned as clients and were seen as individuals with 'deep complicated selves' (Fraser, 2013, p. 73). What was also lost as services for women leaving violence was a shift away from the wider feminist agenda to a welfare service, where the critical links to other needs of women leaving violent relationships, including the need for accessible childcare, a decent income that could support a family and permanent affordable housing were prioritised (Fraser, 2013, p. 72).

Although there is no simple equation between the instrumentalisation of women's services related to domestic violence and the shifts in feminist theoretical framing away from structural analysis of patriarchy towards the post-modern turn, evident in third-way feminisms, there is an intersection with the individualistic nature of that shift and the rise of neoliberalism. Neoliberalism in the West and many other advanced economy nations was highly influential in shifting social discourses and practices away from collective action towards the idealisation of individualism. Acceding to the financial needs of running an organisation or service efficiently and within the corporatised expectations of neoliberal governance, saw women's services silenced and focused on competing for funding. This did not make the problems faced by women go away and based on research we did in Australia with grassroots organisations, it has exacerbated the frustrations felt by frontline workers (mostly feminist advocate providers) dealing with the consequences of domestic violence daily.

What instrumentalisation did was to disarticulate the political objectives of feminist activist providers (Fyall, 2017) of welfare for women in domestic violence services from the potential to influence or change policy. This process was also evident in a study conducted in the UK where researchers examined the differences in approaches between the Scottish and Welsh governments' policy responses to domestic violence services (Charles and MacKay, 2013). In Scotland, with a government highly sympathetic to feminist framing of domestic violence feminist service providers had high-level access to influence policy, whereas in Wales, where the government had been swayed by a purely criminal justice approach, women service providers were disarticulated from policy decisions about resourcing or responding to domestic violence (Charles and MacKay, 2013). In examining the strategies of the women's movement for getting domestic violence on the social policy agenda in South Korea, MinSook Heo found that the way their campaign was framed, to gain public support, had consequences for their feminist agenda, as it ended up reinforcing patriarchal family units:

> The need to disrupt patriarchal discourse about wife beating became tied to the strategic value of calling on certain aspects of the patriarchal family code to draw public support and gain legitimacy for a public agenda that

would include wife beating. At the time, what seemed to be a realistic approach was not considered an obstacle to feminist ideals of helping battered women. It was because of this that the Korean battered women's movement framed the issue as a matter of family breakdown rather than one of male domination. The term "domestic violence" then replaced feminist concepts of "wife beating," "gender violence," or "violence against women" before these concepts had been fully conceptualized and developed. Domestic violence was identified and accepted as an important social problem not because it threatened women with harm, but because it threatened a traditional form of family in Korean society. Given such an understanding of wife battering, it is not surprising that feminist efforts to criminalize marital rape have also confronted institutional and cultural backlash.

(Heo, 2010, p. 231)

Although the historical South Korean experience relates to cultural and political specificity to some extent, it demonstrates a wider challenge for feminist welfare practitioners in keeping pressure on governments to adopt feminist analyses of domestic violence. The most effective means would be to ensure that a government listens to workers on the frontline of domestic violence services, especially in a context of a neoliberal, competitive environment where financial dependency of services becomes a silencing device against advocacy for feminist action and influence. A further challenge is for women to participate in political and governmental spheres, to work towards democracy that embraces collective objectives via pluralist input, opening spaces to listen to frontline workers, feminist activists and people who have experienced domestic violence and ensure that domestic violence is high on political leaderships agendas.

Worldwide Violence against Women

At the time of finalising this book, the world was overtaken by the Coronavirus pandemic. One of the side effects of the pandemic and its subsequent requirement for people to isolate themselves in the confines of their homes for months was the documented rise in the incidence of domestic violence. The combination of an extreme disruption to daily life, continuous presence of all family members in a household and an apparent increase in alcohol and other drug consumption seemed to create a 'perfect' setting for abusers to exercise greater power and perform violence against their intimate partners and other family members. Indeed, the virus threat itself was reported in some cases as another weapon of control:

Still, in recent weeks MRS [Men's Referral Service] staff have seen old tricks take new forms as the pandemic shapes patterns of abuse: men threatening to expose their wives or kids to friends they claim are infected with the virus; men who are even more tightly controlling their partner's movements because they're together all the time; men lashing out when they're stressed about money, or because they disagree with how their partner's parenting their kids, or because they've just lost their job — a common theme counsellors have been picking up on recently.

(Gleeson, 2020)

One way that this surge in domestic violence became evident was through a dramatic increase in searches for domestic violence services on Google and other Internet search engines. There were also reports from the many workers continuing to provide support to people affected by domestic violence, as they had been contacted by telephone on various hotlines. These workers were also frustrated because, due to the confinement laws that had been introduced, they could not provide immediate shelter for people seeking to escape violence (Baird, 2020; Hill, 2019; Gleeson, 2020; Murphy, 2020). In Australia, there were also reports of a dramatic surge in calls to helplines from men, fearful of becoming violent towards their intimate partners (Gleeson, 2020). This apparent pandemic-driven surge in violence against women was occurring worldwide. Initially, it was evident in China during the early period of the pandemic, where it was reported there had been a tripling of incidents of domestic violence (Baird, 2020). There was also an increase in the USA, where, for example, the Seattle Police reported a 20 per cent increase in domestic violence reports in April of 2020 and, in Texas, during March, in the Montgomery County District, there was a 35 per cent increase – both very early in the USA lockdown (Wagers, 2020). It was also reported that the National Domestic Violence Hotline in the USA, had to advise that to be safe, 'women should sleep in their cars to escape violent partners and, during arguments, to stay out of dangerous spaces, such as kitchens and bathrooms' (Fraser, 2020). Other reports indicated that in the UK, domestic abuse killings of women and children increased, doubling the average number of deaths, in Spain an 18 per cent rise in calls to hotlines, in France, police have reported a 30 per cent rise and in Italy, 'hotel rooms had to be requisitioned when shelters were shut down' (Fraser, 2020).

An increase was also evident in Australia as a CEO of a large network of women's refuges reported that 45 per cent of the frontline workers said there had been 'escalating and worsening violence', and 36 per cent said, 'women were reporting violence and abuse related to the COVID-19 crisis (for example, financial or other pressures)' (Baird, 2020). Troublingly, 16 per cent of services reported episodes of 'violence beginning to occur for the first time' (Baird, 2020). The significance of the reported incidences in Australia led the Australian government to make an urgent, special budget allocation for increased domestic violence service availability across the country (Murphy, 2020). The fact that domestic violence, primarily violence against women, was elevated to be one of the key issues during the pandemic indicates its omnipresence and its uniquely domestic nature, exercised between intimate partners and within families.

These are sites that feminists have sought to elevate and illuminate as public concerns, but also sites where relationships, particularly gendered relationships are meant to ensure the welfare of everyday people in everyday life. Hence, feminist practice is the dominant practice for the welfare of women (and their children) experiencing violence at home. This field of practice, probably more than in any other concern of welfare practice, has been extensively researched and has produced a wide range of responses developed by both feminist researchers and practitioners. Despite such intense focus, it remains one of the most obvious threats to the welfare of women and children across the world.

In the broadest sense, domestic violence is defined as:

> … any act of gender-based violence that results in, or is likely to result in, physical, sexual, or mental harm or suffering to women, including threats of such acts, coercion, or arbitrary deprivation of liberty, whether occurring in public or in private life.
>
> *(United Nations, 1993)*

An Ongoing Global Problem

Violence against women is a pervasive and persistent global problem (Weldon and Htun, 2013). More than 35 per cent of women worldwide, which is around 818 million women, almost the total population of sub-Saharan Africa and almost three times the population of the USA, have experienced either physical, or sexual, partner violence or non-partner sexual violence (Klugman et al., 2014; WHO, 2021). The United Nations Office of Drugs and Crime reported that an estimated 87,000 women were killed around the world in 2017, 58 per cent (50,000 women) by intimate partners or family members. This equates to 1.3 victims per 100,000 of the female population around the world, six women being killed every hour by people they know (UNODC, 2018). As noted in Chapter 2, the United Nations Sustainable Development Goal, Goal 5, Gender Inequality has as its second target 'Eliminate all forms of violence against all women and girls in the public and private spheres, including trafficking and sexual and other types of exploitation' (UN SDGs, 2016). Researchers tend to agree that the objectives of this target have not been met and in fact, there has been an increase in the incidence of domestic violence worldwide (Leight, 2022).

The death of women at the hand of a violent partner or ex-partner is of course an extreme outcome of violence against women but reinforces the gendered nature of domestic violence. The extent of gendered violence against women in the contemporary world is one of the strongest indicators that efforts by social movements, global institutions and states have been largely unsuccessful at overcoming traditionally informed views of gender inequality. This is despite universal agreements between women from many nations via the Fourth World Conference on Women in Beijing in 1995, where a platform for action defined violence against women, called upon states to act against violence against women, and established the Convention on the Elimination of All Forms of Discrimination against Women (CEDAW) (UN Women, 2000). Since then, there have been several efforts on a global scale to work towards gender equality and address violence against women. However, it is in the recently declared United Nations Sustainable Development Goals that we have seen a comprehensive acknowledgement that women's inequality cannot be overcome without addressing violence against women at systemic and interpersonal levels (UN SDGs, 2016).

In writing about violence against women in India, Samta Pandya observed that due to cultural, religious, and traditional constructions of female sexuality in India "women are subjected to rape, female circumcision/genital mutilation, female infanticide and sex-related crimes. Due to dependence on men and relationships with a man/men, women are vulnerable to domestic violence" (2014, p. 501). Further, although dowries have been illegal in India since 1961, dowry-related deaths and violence are still widespread, for example in 2015 a total of 24,771 dowry deaths and 348,000 cases of 'cruelty by a husband to a relative' were reported in India over the prior three years (India Express, 2015). Another gendered violent practice that governments have legislated against is honour killings. This practice, of families killing or instigating killings of a female family member as a matter of honour, is widespread in the Middle East and North Africa and, due to migration from many countries in those regions, it also occurs amongst diasporas in the USA, the UK, Canada and Europe (Kulczycki and Windle, 2011). Honour killings

> are perpetrated for a range of offenses related to the perceived misuse of female sexuality, most notably marital infidelity and premarital sex. Unacceptable behaviours may also include contacting persons of different faiths, initiating a separation or divorce, being a victim of rape, and even such alleged misdemeanours as flirting, or otherwise impugning the family honour.
>
> *(Kulczycki and Windle, 2011, p. 1443)*

Kulczycki and Windle drew the following conclusions after a wide analysis of research on honour killings:

> The primary reasons why honour killings are seen to occur in the patriarchal and patrilineal societies of the MENA [*Middle East and Africa*] region is because they are a mechanism for maintaining strict control over women, their reproductive power, and designated familial power structures. Honour killings remove potentially aberrant behaviour from the system and provide an example to others who might deviate from the norm. The state apparatus reproduces and effectively reinforces the entrenched patriarchal and other socio-cultural attitudes that give rise to these violent acts. It has little need to disrupt the patriarchal system, and the private, familial context of honour killings serves as a pretext for non-intervention.
>
> *(2011, p. 1455)*

The above analysis makes important links between the structure of a patriarchal society and the systemic oppression of women, which, as feminists have observed since the second wave, also imposes oppressive masculine expectations and restrictions on men. It highlights the danger of excluding the private, domestic sphere from public responsibility, out of sight of policy makers and criminal justice systems. Like many forms of violence against women, this is a critical issue for feminist practice within specific cultures as well as across cultures. As ethnic traditions of women's systematic oppression can and are carried into non-traditional societies through migration, ethnically supported violence requires a practice response at diverse sites.

A first step in countering violence and acting in solidarity with women and girls who face or have experienced systemic cultural oppressions is to grasp an understanding of how power is exercised and perpetuated to maintain control over women and others deemed of a lesser status than those who hold power in relationships. This often requires challenges to arguments of cultural specificity and, in practice, demands decisions that prioritise one ethical position over other views that argue tradition and culture as reasons for certain practices. From a feminist perspective, the fundamental position would be to challenge any practice or belief that oppresses or harms women because they *are* women but, basing the challenge on accepting differences learned from the knowledge and experiences of the women within any specific cultural context. This is a critical point for feminist practice. Lila Abu-Lughod put forward a clear perspective on the tensions for outsider feminist attempts to 'rescue' women from perceived oppressive cultural practices:

> ... might other desires be more meaningful for different groups of people? Living in close families? Living in a godly way? Living without war? I have done fieldwork in Egypt over more than twenty years and cannot think of a single woman I know, from the poorest rural to the most educated cosmopolitan, who has ever expressed envy of US women, women they tend to perceive as bereft of community, vulnerable to sexual violence and social anomie or strangely disrespectful of God.
>
> *(2002, p. 788)*

Abu-Lughod emphasised that this is not cultural relativism, where culture can excuse certain practices, but rather it involves the hard work of 'recognising and respecting differences' that should be seen as 'expressions of different circumstances and as manifestations of differently structured desires', including different ideas of justice and personhood (2002, pp. 787–788). These ideas are not limited to international comparisons as in settler nations such as Australia, the USA and Canada, similar issues arise in feminist practice in social welfare and domestic violence in Indigenous communities within those countries. In such cases, colonial impositions that assert culture by the colonisers have already systematically denied difference and imposed cultural and social norms through various forms of structural violence (racism-informed justice responses, for example).

In Latin America violence against women has extended well beyond the domestic sphere, where 'Mexican and Central American women's organisations use the term *femicidio* as a legal and political term to refer to the murder of women killed *because they are women*' (Prieto-Carrón et al., 2007; The Economist, 2020). Based on this definition, *femicido* has, since 2007, become a legally recognised category of killing in 15 Latin American countries, although the concept of how victims experience their deaths varies from country to country (The Economist, 2020). In Mexico, the phenomenon of *femicido* includes domestic violence, women being killed by their intimate partners. In 2019, 1,006 murders in Mexico were classified as femicides and many of the victims had been raped, mutilated, and dumped. In response, Mexican women organised protests of tens of thousands of women and a national strike, refusing to go to work or do any domestic chores, to bring attention to the crisis (Phillips, 2022; Villegas, 2020). In response to large, angry street protests some specialist police units were established, Femicide Units. Many of the units were under-resourced and ineffectual at finding the perpetrators. However, the unit in Mexico City was coordinated by a feminist human rights lawyer, Sayuri Herrera, who had women on the police team investigating deaths and others working with her to solve 700 previous killings that the police had conveniently labelled as suicides, reflecting a callous disregard for the level of domestic violence in Mexican society as well as a complicity by many male police tasked with investigating the crimes (Ferguson and Henry, 2022). Other activists were frustrated that even though there was a left-wing government in Mexico the number of women being killed continued to rise with a rate of ten or 11 women killed per day (Phillips, 2022). Salguero, one feminist activist, created a web-based map of where the murders had taken place and recorded regular details of the murders. By March 2022 she had logged 320 deaths, and from the time of creating the map in January 2016, she has recorded more than 9,000 deaths (Phillips, 2022).

Brazil had the fifth highest rate of femicides in South America. There were also 54,000 victims of rape and 263,000 cases of women injured due to domestic violence in 2018 (Targeted News Service, 2020). This level of violence in Brazil has occurred under an extreme right-wing government led by President Bolsonaro, which reduced the funding for the Women's Secretariat that managed a program to support victims, from US$25 million in 2015 to US$1.1 million in 2019 (Targeted News Service, 2020). In a country with extreme economic inequality, where gender pay inequity and racism (black women earn less than half of the average income of white men) makes black women highly vulnerable to violence, where any rise in violence against women is generally against black women (Targeted News Service, 2020).

Population-level surveys based on reports from victims provide the most accurate estimates of the prevalence of intimate partner violence and sexual violence in non-conflict (non-war) settings. The most extensive research conducted on the incidence of domestic violence was carried out in a multi-country study conducted by the World Health Organisation in 2004. The study was developed in cooperation with women's organisations, and this was reflected in the clearly feminist approach and implementation of the study. The study required the voices of women to inform the study rather than relying on criminal statistics or reporting data. Interviews were conducted with '24,000 women from 15 sites in ten countries representing diverse cultural settings: Bangladesh, Brazil, Ethiopia, Japan, Namibia, Peru, Samoa, Serbia and Montenegro, Thailand, and the United Republic of Tanzania' (WHO, 2005). The study found that among women aged 15–49:

- between 15% of women in Japan and 71% of women in Ethiopia reported physical and/or sexual violence by an intimate partner in their lifetime
- between 0.3 and 11.5% of women reported sexual violence by someone other than a partner since the age of 15 years
- the first sexual experience for many women was reported as forced – 17% of women in rural Tanzania, 24% in rural Peru and 30% in rural Bangladesh reported that their first sexual experience was forced.

(WHO, 2005).

The WHO study demonstrates the extensive incidence of violence against women across the world and markedly reflects that in countries with lower economic wealth the incidence or experience of violence for women and girls is evidently greater. The report found that

> the proportion of women who had ever suffered physical violence by a male partner ranged from 13 per cent in Japan to 61 per cent in provincial Peru. Japan also had the lowest level of sexual violence at 6 per cent, with the highest figure of 59 per cent being reported in Ethiopia.
>
> *(WHO, 2005, p. 6)*

This demonstrates how economic class can be a critical intersection with gender and ethnicity, as it could be argued that the broader construct of patriarchy is not that different in economically wealthy Japan compared to economically poor Thailand or Peru. It is also arguable that in higher socioeconomic groupings within richer countries, violence against women is more hidden and women can be more isolated in lower-density communities. Legal processes to protect women from sexual assault are very limited in Japan and in a culture that has a glorification of eroticised violence, women's capacity to use the law for protection and justice is very limited and highly prejudicial (Burns, 2013, p. 6). It was not until 2002 that there was any law that could be used to protect women from their violent partners and was introduced into a culture that was complicit in hiding violence against women:

> For many years in Japan, domestic violence existed in the shadows—it was a husband's prerogative, a private family matter. Finally, a law gives women

some protections, but the burden of proof is on women and abuse is still not a crime.

(Rice, 2001)

Rice (2001) noted that the new law did not actually make domestic abuse a crime due to patriarchal traditions in Japan where men's superiority to women supported men's violence in the domestic sphere, with no role for criminal justice or policing. In analysing the context of the new laws, Honda and Ogawa (2021) pointed out that global women's movement events such as the UN Convention on CEDAW (ratified by Japan in 1985) had been pivotal in the Japanese women's movement setting up refuges for domestic violence victims. However widespread support and reform have been difficult. They also reported that there had been a dramatic uptake in counselling and support services since the introduction of the Bill but that the number of incidences filed with police continues to rise, reaching over 80,000 in 2019 (Honda and Ogawa, 2021). Consistent with a feminist analysis, Honda and Ogawa, after analysing a wide variety of books about domestic violence, available to the public, concluded that it was 'necessary to provide a clear explanation of domestic violence as a problem that takes place within the context of gender-inequal society' and where offenders, seek to exercise 'absolute control over their partners' (2021, p. 42). Forcing governments to create and implement laws and appropriate services is a powerful part of feminist practice, as is the ongoing battle for gender equality through promoting an understanding of it as an underlying cause of gendered violence.

Feminist activists were able to finally get a Domestic Violence Prevention Act introduced in Taiwan, in 1998, after two high-profile incidents that gained wide public attention, including the murder of a women's rights activist (Kuan, 2021). This made it the first country in Asia to create a comprehensive law relating to all aspects of domestic violence, including a focus on criminality of acts of violence, safety for women and prevention strategies (Kuan, 2021). Kuan noted:

> Similar to other cultures in the world, the patriarchal Chinese tradition used to deem violence in the family as a family matter and was excluded from the state's scrutiny and intervention. Before the enactment of DVP Act, the laws gave victims of domestic violence access to legal remedies aftermath in a civil suit, filed for a divorce, or filed assault complaints pursuant to the criminal procedure. However, the enforcement of such law was hamstrung by the traditional ideology of "family domain shall be free from the legal intervention (法不入家門)" and "even an upright official finds it hard to settle a family quarrel (清官難斷家務事)".
>
> *(2021, p. 25)*

The family was for hundreds of years a law-free zone in Taiwan, which left victims of domestic violence helpless and powerless (Chen, 2013, p. 45). The mechanisms put in place in Taiwan that arose from the law being introduced in 1998 have resulted in an extensive and well-known hotline service and have reached children and migrant women (Kuan, 2021). However, Kuan (2021) noted that domestic violence prevalence is still high in Taiwan and that women experiencing domestic violence with intersectional issues such as poverty, disability, and older age, for example, are overlooked. In her analysis of the current context, Kuan argued for a larger focus on gender inequality, as an underlying cause of gender-based violence against women as the current high incidence 'reflects the fact that gender stereotypes and misogyny continue to perpetuate Taiwanese society and family' (2021, p. 33).

As can be noted from the examples of legislative change across the world, contemporary feminist practice is a critical frontline in the struggle to end violence against women. Despite it being generally now accepted as a core social policy responsibility of the state that must be addressed through legislation, policing and criminal intervention, public education and specific services, the continued prevalence of domestic violence is overwhelming. Based on a global study conducted in 2018, Sardinha et al., made the following observation:

> It is important to note that there are 28 countries within the past year [2018] where physical or sexual, or both, intimate partner violence prevalence is substantially higher than the global average. Several of these are countries were affected by conflict. These findings are consistent with the different social, economic, and political circumstances that are associated with intimate partner violence and limit women's ability to leave abusive relationships, such as economic insecurity, gender inequitable norms, high amounts of societal stigma, economic insecurity, discriminatory family law, and inadequate support services.
>
> *(2022, p. 811)*

The intersectionality of race, gender and economic status, and the risk of violence is stark in many contexts, for example, but it is a common factor across the world, as having access to resources to escape domestic violence is a key component of women's safety, for both immediate and longer-term needs. It is for this reason that gender equality is necessarily linked to violence against women in any strategies aimed at welfare for women in any society.

Why Is There Still Such Violence against Women Worldwide and How Is It Countered?

Perpetual acts of violence against women appear to be an insoluble policy and practice problem in wider society, and for women's social welfare. Given the now lengthy history of feminist activism, program development, practical interventions and services by feminist practitioners, the enormous investments in attempts to address the underlying causes and bases of violence against women, we appear to be no closer to changing the gender power relations that underpin such violence. For those working to support women who have experienced violence from intimate partners, who advocate for and provide safety for women and their children and those who seek to educate men and change their violent behaviour towards women, the overall gains seem small. There is one argument that suggests that the level of incidence of domestic violence has not changed, rather it is now more visible owing to higher levels of public awareness and justice responses by the state. For welfare practitioners, this is unhelpful and fails to recognise that public awareness does not appear to be married to public responsibility or social justice related to inequality. Of course, in some countries, the state has not made domestic violence illegal. In Iran for example there are no laws that recognise domestic violence as a crime despite research showing its high prevalence (Nikparvar et al., 2021). Research on incidence in Iran found that 48 per cent of women in the study (*n* 702) had experienced violence from their intimate partner (Nikparvar et al., 2021). Despite the wider culture creating strict taboos about women leaving a marriage under any circumstances, there are some government-funded refuges in Iran, although their presence is not widely known (Nikparvar et al., 2021).

There are many tensions between the involvement of and reliance on the state (on governments) in both justice interventions through the criminalisation of domestic violence and feminist interventions for policy that seeks to change gender power relations. Such tensions are deeply rooted in historical relations between the state and women's oppression. The history of such relationships is recent and still present in some countries where instruments of the state (for example, the police and discriminatory laws related to labour rights, family, political power, and property) reflect the overall masculinised framework of a society. Research on how domestic and sexual violence are framed by the law and endorsed by political action or inaction have shown that solutions to the 'problem' of domestic violence are elusive. In MinSook Heo's research on domestic violence legislation in South Korea, mentioned previously, she also observed that:

> Korean feminists have realized that state engagement *per se* does not guarantee the political influence of the women's movement on state policy. Instead, state intervention led to a discontinuation of movement influence. It was feminists who identified the problem of domestic violence and who helped draft the very Acts that have resulted in their marginalization and disempowerment.
>
> *(2010, p. xx)*

In a study of 70 countries' domestic violence policy responses over 30 years, Weldon and Htun (2013) found the most important factor that ensured government action, including legal reform, public education campaigns, and women's safety measures, was feminist activism. Weldon's (2002) previous research also found that the number of women in government, and pluralist democratic governance were key factors. Pluralist democracies allow 'seats at the table', or ministerial access, to represent the interests of social movements, minority interests and civil society in developing policy responses to social or economic problems.

What hasn't been widely accounted for is the question of what inhibits the kind of social transformation that would result in gender equality and the end of targeted violence within the domestic sphere. Accountability is a core aspect of responding to male violence against women. For centuries, the law has generally held people to account for violence they inflict on others, especially in the public sphere, but the responsibility of those who stand by and allow violence to occur is a less clear field of accountability. The following extract from a news report of a specific case of domestic violence is a demonstration that explains how 'causes' go well beyond singular acts by singular men:

> Three weeks of torture and repeated sexual assaults, a victim on the brink of death, a sadistic banker lurking in a swanky suburb, and a desperate police manhunt culminating in a dramatic car chase.
>
> The evidence tendered at the sentencing hearing of Nicholas Crilley, in Brisbane this week, reads like the screenplay of a hit American crime show. Maybe that's the problem. Perhaps we prefer to pretend this isn't real. Because right now, it almost beggars belief that Australian women are dying regularly in such horrific circumstances and we are not marching on the streets, demanding change... the swank riverside suburb of Bulimba, where Crilley, now 34, had held his former girlfriend against her will in a townhouse in 2017. "I've pummelled her so hard ... she can't talk anymore," he boasted to a friend during his rampage.
>
> Crilley had told the then 21-year-old victim he intended to "disfigure her face" and break her jaw, but he went much further than that. When police eventually located the young woman, they thought at first that she was dead, the likely victim of an explosion. But the life-threatening burns covering almost half her body had been caused by Crilley, who had poured boiling water on her, and then acetone, before setting her on fire. ...[He] had also broken her nose, sternum, ribs, cheekbone and one eye socket, and gouged a hole in the side of her head "most likely caused by a screwdriver or similar", the court was told. Crilley would often pause during the assaults to photograph or film the injuries he had caused. Ultimately, he would be charged with more than 50 separate offences. His housemate was also charged. He had not caused injuries, but nor had he intervened to protect the seriously injured woman, or to alert authorities.
>
> (Jackman, 2020)

This was a case where the complicity of the other man in the household was recognised and acted on. In another incidence of domestic violence in Australia, by an ex-partner, a woman was murdered in her home, and police reported that over several hours, neighbours heard screams and cries for help, including a scream stating that 'he is going to kill me' and yet nobody acted to intervene or call the police (South Australian Police, 2020). The complicity of a man living in the same house while another man tortured and killed a woman and neighbours who failed to act to protect a woman from being murdered reflects the idea that men's violence towards women with whom they are in or had a relationship with is socially tolerable and acceptable. It infers that it is a private matter and reflects an acceptance that men can assert control and power over women in the domestic sphere. This complicity is similar to the agreement amongst men to sexually assault women, to threaten women in social media, to act out any form of aggression and control that is known amongst men and emerges as a shared goal to maintain their sense of power. It is very common that the domestic nature of domestic violence absolves those around such offences from any intervention or action.

Government action is dominated by criminalising responses that focus on the offender, which once in the justice system, the process loses touch with the wider social collusion that gives license to such acts and rarely demands that a perpetrator demonstrates a sense of accountability for his actions. Although there have been many programs aimed at changing men's violent behaviour toward women, aiming at making them accountable, significant changes appear to be rare, unless men stay in lengthy programs (see Arce et al., 2020 for example). The other large investment is in public and school education campaigns that also tend to focus on one-to-one relationships. Young people are told to respect their partner but not necessarily intervene, ask hard questions or prevent actions taken by those around them or indeed how to counter the violence of toxic masculinity that surrounds them in popular culture and sport, for example. Men are told that domestic violence is not acceptable and to speak of their friend's actions but are not told to report their friends who humiliate, hurt, and control their intimate partners to police. There are other widely circulating public discourses that work against the feminist analysis of domestic violence and men's accountability. One is the Australian men's movement generated argument that one in three victims of domestic violence are men (Oneinthree, 2020), which seeks to bring a focus on men as victims and criticise government campaigns against men's violence against women. This type of activity can of course be important for men who have experienced domestic violence at the hands of women partners and men in same-sex relationships who have experienced such violence, but it cannot be used to deny the overwhelming dominance of violence against women and the requirement for men to be held to account. The other widely reported discourse that seemed to emerge in the first instance of media reporting on domestic violence-related homicides is that the perpetrator was a good person and must have been stressed, depressed, or pushed to take such action. Often generated in media reports by surprised neighbours and friends, there is a narrative that seeks to find a reason beyond the perpetrator's immediate actions. Extensive research by the Australian network Our Watch, on 152 deaths sought to address the 'myth' that men who kill their partner and sometimes their children 'just snap' and commit terrible acts of violence. They reported that:

> This report tells us the powerful story behind these figures. Information was collected from the Coroner's Courts, police investigations, court proceedings and inquest findings.
>
> The network's research showed that men commit more than 80 per cent of murders in couples with a history of domestic violence. The overwhelming majority of those men had a history of abusing the women they ultimately killed.
>
> Distressingly, more than one-third of the murders were committed by men occurred after the relationship had ended and nearly a quarter of the women killed had Domestic Violence Orders against their killer at the time of the murder.
>
> *(Kinnersly, 2018)*

Accountability can take a range of forms, apart from the obvious need for perpetrators to be accountable for their actions. Everyone in a community must also take responsibility for what is happening next door, in their neighbourhood, amongst their friends. The apparently deeply entrenched notion of what happens in the private sphere of the home is a private matter has been consistently challenged by feminist activism related to domestic violence, sexual assault and child abuse and must be part of wider campaigns for public understanding; in this sense, everyone is accountable for domestic violence.

Understanding Domestic Violence Research

In Australia, criminology statistics confirm that women are the most likely victims of 'domestic/family' homicides. This was demonstrated in a study that analysed data over a ten-year period from 2002 to 2012, which revealed that 60 per cent of domestic/family homicides were female and 75 per cent of those were victims of domestic violence (Cussen and Bryan, 2015). As noted in the above international context, femicide data is important because it is undeniable and more reliable than data on the overall incidence of domestic violence, which includes physical, emotional and financial acts of control within intimate relationships, as such incidents of violence are notoriously under-reported. There is, however, extensive research data on the experience of the various forms of violence and criminal statistics on (physical) 'domestic assault' or domestic abuse crimes. UK research on experiences of intimate partner abuse showed that twice as many women as men between the ages of 16 years and 59 years had reported 'experiencing any type of domestic abuse in the last year' that is, 'partner / ex-partner abuse (non-sexual), family abuse (non-sexual) and sexual assault or stalking carried out by a current or former partner or other family member' (ONS, 2016). This is equivalent to an estimated 1.3 million female victims and

600,000 male victims (ONS, 2016). However, as there is a strong backlash from some men (often organised in men's rights groups in Australia, the USA and the UK) to the representation of domestic violence/abuse as being a crime primarily against women, it is important to understand the complexity of much of the data collected on domestic violence. In the UK data, even though the research showed almost equal numbers of men as women stating they had experienced force in domestic abuse, the severity of abuse is starkly differentiated when the severity of injuries due to abuse is considered. For example, based on data

> for the year ending March 2013 to the year ending March 2015, additional analysis was carried out on victims who received medical attention. It was found that of those victims who received medical attention, 73 per cent were female and 27 per cent were male.
>
> *(ONS, 2016)*

This level of detail is important from a feminist perspective when counteracting claims from men's rights groups that claim that they are equally victims of domestic violence.

Data is also available on incidents of domestic assaults responded to by police that tend to relate to physical violence. For example, the New South Wales Bureau of Crime Statistics and Research (NSWBCSR) (2016) mapped the incidence via local government regions across the state of New South Wales (NSW) in Australia, with the data demonstrating that the areas of high incidence of domestic assaults were also areas of high socio-economic disadvantage. Reported domestic violence in the worst area of NSW was 1,138 per 100,000 (NSWBCSR, 2016). A feminist analysis of such data might observe that women who live in low socio-economic circumstances have less capacity and resources to escape violent relationships due to the lack of immediate respite and longer-term issues such as no realistic childcare options, work options or educational opportunities, all deeply structural, socio-economic and geographical barriers to choosing independence.

To ensure that the social welfare issue of domestic violence is kept in the public sphere, some Australian feminist activists have acted to ensure that when a woman has been murdered by a violent partner or family member she is immediately recognised as a victim of domestic violence. This has been a political strategy to highlight the extent of domestic violence by a social media activist group called 'Destroy the Joint', which publicises an ongoing tally of the number of women murdered by their current or past intimate partner (Destroy the Joint, 2022). The data presented is based on immediate reporting of deaths and the research done by journalists into that reporting. This provides a current statistical account that is not based on waiting for criminal justice processes or coroner's findings, which allows for an immediate tally. For example, in 2016, 73, in 2019, 62, in 2020, 69 in 2021, 53 women had been killed in Australia in domestic situations (Destroy the Joint, 2022). Each reported death is detailed and made available on the Destroy the Joint Facebook page. The tally project has been successful in keeping the incidence of deaths from domestic violence on the political and public agendas as the tally is often cited as a deeply troubling statistic of more than one woman per week dying at the hands of a current or past partner or relative. However, the Destroy the Joint activist feminists who run the social media site also use it as a tool for creating intersections between all key issues of concern to feminists, effectively using social media to critique acts of misogyny and sexism occurring in public life (Destroy the Joint, 2022).

Social work, legal, sociological, political, psychological and health research on domestic violence is extensive. It ranges from building knowledge about it as a lived experience, to exploring its criminality, social construction, role in gender inequality, nature, impact and as a pathology. Research that explores the experience of domestic violence has led to important, deep understandings of how to detect and recognise what may be happening in some intimate relationships and its long-term impact on survivors and their children (Douglas and Walsh, 2010; Hill, 2019; Holland et al., 2018; Katz, 2019; Namy et al., 2017; Stark, 2007; Tsantefski et al., 2018). The number of very specific ways that men abuse women through coercive control, physical, emotional and financial violence, threats, and intimidation has been extensively documented. For example, it has been determined that men also use reproductive control as a form of violence against women. Lévesque et al. (2020) found that men in shorter-term relationships subverted women's wishes to have children and in long-term relationships used this form of violence to force their partners to get pregnant against their wishes. Feminist researchers have also sought to understand how domestic violence is reflected in 'relational power' within family households. In a rare study of domestic violence in family households in Kampala, Uganda researchers found, among other factors, widely accepted levels of physical disciplining in violence against children, which related to violence against their mothers in two ways, that the male partner's violence against them prompted women to exercise 'displaced aggression' on their children and that the father's violence against their children caused emotional violence against mothers through 'bystander trauma' (Namy et al., 2017). Analysis in this study was closely linked to a wider, structural framework established by the researchers:

> … such dynamics cannot be divorced from women's systemic oppression and their relational power within the family. Thus, within a highly constrained environment, women may violently express their powerlessness – or attempt to consolidate their own power – over children, who are perceived as subordinate within the hierarchy.
>
> *(Namy et al., 2017, p. 47)*

From a social welfare practice perspective, such findings urge a complex, deeper understanding of the mothers' actions in this context, where violence against children is normalised and accepted in the wider social culture but violence against women is not seen in the same way, despite its high level of incidence and a tendency to attribute men's violence to normative, hegemonic masculinity in the strongly patriarchal Ugandan culture (Hundle, 2019). The study was intent on revealing how assertions of power manifest in harm to both children and mothers due to gender inequality more broadly. However, despite the conclusion that the violence that took place within families related to the hierarchy within the family, it did appear that external public discourse and legislative action against violence against women had influenced views about domestic violence, seeing it as less acceptable than violence against children (Namy et al., 2017, p. 47).

Despite extensive research data representing an apparently indisputable social problem, violence against women remains controversial and despite social progress towards greater gender equality in many countries, violence against women by their intimate partners and relatives continues to be one of the most common crimes committed every day, everywhere. Substantial research on services, interventions and incidences of domestic violence that provide ample evidence of its existence and its gendered nature has not resulted in an uncontested domain. In fact, due to its very nature, it has been subjected to many contradictory often deeply felt and argued differences. Debates about domestic violence have taken place in every sphere. There are debates in scholarship and research, in the popular media, within governments amongst politicians and policymakers and within professional (health, mental health, legal, policing, psychiatric and social work) and community services that have been established to address, combat, respond to and advocate around domestic violence. Even the term domestic violence is controversial as, depending on political, cultural and ideological perspectives, it has been described as family violence, violence against women, gender-based violence, interpersonal violence, spousal violence, wife bashing, battered women and so on. However, its recognition as a social policy problem as well as a societal problem is entirely due to the efforts of feminist activists who fought to bring it out into the open. It is the juxtaposition between the intimate partner violence taking place in the domestic sphere, which had previously been seen as private spaces where there should not be public scrutiny of behaviour, and the wider concerns of violence in the community where laws usually protect people from systematic violence against strangers, that the term *domestic* violence was chosen by feminist activists. The term required a public sphere view and response to what could not remain a private problem in the domestic sphere. This was also an important challenge to pathologising discourses that saw domestic violence as a mental illness or deviance in men (and other offenders), rather than a deep-seated privilege of men exercising patriarchal power over those seen as less equal.

Health and Domestic Violence

Another area of importance in social and medical research is the effects of domestic violence on women's health and its impact on practice. Early second-wave feminists such as Phyllis Chesler (1972), established connections between documented higher rates of mental illness in women and the powerful impact of patriarchy and misogyny. Chesler (1972) observed that patriarchy determined how women would be seen and treated for mental illness, and that views of mental illness were determined by a patriarchal construction of what it was to be a woman, of 'femininity'. She also noted that in seeking help for mental illness, women would be confronted with an entirely male-run system, medical professionals and hospitals were completely controlled by a patriarchal framework and by men (Chesler, 1972). Since then, many more women are involved in practices that assist and support women and feminist social work researchers have established and documented the connections between the incidence of women's poor mental well-being and domestic violence (Humphreys and Thiara, 2003; Moulding, 2016a, 2016b).

Collaboration between feminist researchers and medical professionals in hospitals has resulted in automatic screening procedures for domestic violence and heightened awareness of the mental health effects of domestic violence (Laing, 2003; Laing et al., 2012). However, despite extensive investment in research on acquired brain injuries for football players and other athletes, a lot less has occurred for women who sustain traumatic/acquired brain injuries (TBIs) from domestic violence. USA-based researchers, Costello and Greenwald (2022) observed that it is only since the 1990s that medical research into the relationship between domestic violence and traumatic or acquired brain injury has emerged resulting in it being only recently understood. They also observed that it is 'estimated that the number of women who have experienced TBI secondary to domestic violence is 11–12 times greater than the number of TBIs experienced by military personnel and athletes combined' (Costello and Greenwald, 2022). According to brain injury research, domestic violence causes brain injury 'through aggressive shaking, strangulation, a blow to the head (with a fist and/or heavy object) and falling/being thrown to the floor' (Costello and Greenwald, 2022).

In a study with domestic violence service practitioners, Ayton et al. (2021) found that practitioners believed 30 to 40 per cent of women using their service had brain injuries from the violence they had experienced. The implications of such injuries are significant and long lasting but are under-reported or not understood in line with the overall underreporting of incidences of domestic violence. Medical research has found that by the time a woman has escaped the violent relationship she is likely to have experienced extensive, repeated trauma to the brain. Various studies concluded that there was a general lack of awareness and understanding of traumatic (acquired) brain injury and its symptoms among domestic violence service providers (Ayton et al., 2021; Haag, 2019; Nemeth et al., 2019). An Australian study also explored the connection between perpetrators of domestic violence with acquired brain injury who had encountered the criminal justice system and concluded that more research and understanding of acquired brain injured perpetrators and victims was required (Lansdell et al., 2021).

Apart from emphasising the ongoing trauma of experiencing domestic violence, these types of studies are valuable for feminist practitioners advocating to address research gaps, promote professional and public education, and develop aspects in services to ensure women suffering brain injuries get appropriate treatment and support (Lansdell et al., 2021; Nemeth et al., 2019). One suggestion for practitioners is to introduce screening questionnaires that allow for indicators of brain injury so that appropriate medical referrals can be made. At the very least, practitioners should be informed about common physical symptoms so that medical referrals can be made. These include headaches, fatigue, sleep disturbances, vertigo, and pain and cognitive symptoms can be seen to affect attention, concentration, and executive functioning (Haag et al., 2019). This wide array of potential health effects can create risk situations for women with children as well as risks to their custody and care of children, making awareness of them as side effects from domestic violence critical in many service contexts.

Conclusion

In this chapter the social welfare of women and their children who have experienced or are experiencing domestic violence has been the focus. Understanding the widespread nature of violence against women across the world is an important aspect of knowledge in this field of social welfare practice, as it informs social policy and service responses. Examples of feminist responses, particularly activism towards establishing or reforming laws and services, in different national and cultural contexts have been drawn upon to generate diverse perspectives on how feminists have sought to address widespread acts of violence against women. The role of the state has also been a focus, as the way in which domestic violence is framed by the state has a deep impact on the criminal justice system and resources for women's safety.

Although domestic violence has been the specific focus of this chapter other forms of gendered violence have also been acknowledged, systematic forms of violence that are culturally sanctioned. Rape, femicide and other forms of sexual abuse are connected because the violence occurs against women because they are women. The focus on men as perpetrators of this widespread violence relates to a world where gender inequality is still deeply entrenched. Some feminists argue against broad generalisations of women's experience of violence, however extensive research that includes many voices of women across the world involved in attempts to eliminate domestic violence attests to the unified objectives of feminist practice in social welfare related to the safety of and justice for women affected by domestic violence.

At the beginning of this chapter, I raised some key questions for consideration. The answers are directly and indirectly addressed throughout the chapter, but largely point to the importance of the sustainability of the key factors that lead to greater accountability of governments and communities for the violence against women that takes place every day in the domestic sphere. Consistent with the broader themes in this book, feminist practice is political practice and must engage with every level of political action, the personal, the community, the public sphere, and each level of government. There is ample evidence that feminist practitioners are doing this across the world in their efforts to address the incidence and impact of domestic violence but wider social transformations that lead to gender equality are key to the sustainability of efforts to eliminate violence against women.

References

Abu-Lughod, L. (2002) Do Muslim women really need saving? Anthropological reflections on cultural relativism and its others. *American Anthropologist*, 104 (3), 783–790.

Arce, R., Arias, E., Novo, M. and Fariña, F. (2020) Are interventions with batterers effective? A meta-analytical review. *Psychosocial Intervention*, 29 (3), 153–164.

Ayton, D., Pritchard, E. and Tsindos, T. (2021) Acquired brain injury in the context of family violence: A systematic scoping review of incidence, prevalence, and contributing factors. *Trauma, Violence, & Abuse*, 22 (1), 3–17.

Baird, J. (2020) When isolating at home becomes a danger to life. *The Sydney Morning Herald*, March 28, 2020. (Accessed March 31, 2020). https://www.smh.com.au/national/when-isolating-at-home-becomes-a-danger-to-life-20200327-p54ejx.html.

Bowstead, J.C. (2015). Why women's domestic violence refuges are not local services. *Critical Social Policy*, 35 (3), 327–349.

Burns, C. (2013) *Sexual Violence and Law in Japan*. London: Routledge.

Charles, N. and MacKay, F. (2013) Feminist politics and framing contests: Domestic violence policy in Scotland and Wales. *Critical Social Policy*, 33 (4), 593–615.

Chen, H. (2013) Gender mainstreaming and the protection of women's personal safety: Beginning with the experience in Taiwan. *Private Law*, 21, 41–67.

Chesler, P. (1972) *Women and Madness* (1st ed.). Garden City, NY: Doubleday.

Costello, K. and Greenwald, B.D. (2022) Update on domestic violence and traumatic brain injury: A narrative review. *Brain Sciences*, 12 (1), 122.

Cussen, T. and W. Bryan (2015) Domestic/family homicide in Australia. *Research in Practice*. No. 38. Canberra: Australian Institute of Criminology, Australian Government. http://www.aic.gov.au/media_library/publications/rip/rip38/rip38.pdf.

Destroy the Joint (2022) Counting dead women Australia 2022. We count every known death due to violence against women in Australia. (Accessed March 9, 2022). https://www.facebook.com/Counting-Dead-Women-Australia-111647810713234/.

Douglas, H. and Walsh, T. (2010). Mothers, domestic violence, and child protection. *Violence against Women*, 16 (5), 489–508.

Ferguson, S. and Henry, M. (2022) She was facing a real monster. *Foreign Correspondent*. Australian Broadcasting Commission (ABC), March 25, 2022. https://www.abc.net.au/news/2022-03-24/mexico-femicide-units-violent-crime-women-foreign-correspondent/100920716.

Fraser, C. (2020) When will we care about domestic violence? *New York Review*, May 28, 2020, Issue. https://www.nybooks.com/articles/2020/05/28/when-will-we-care-about-domestic-violence/.

Fraser, N. (2013). *Fortunes of Feminism, from State Managed Capitalism to Neoliberal Crisis*. London; Brooklyn, NY: Verso.

Fyall, R. (2017) Nonprofits as advocates and providers: A conceptual framework. *Policy Studies Journal*, 45 (1) 121–143.

Garg, S., Singh, M.M., Rustagi, R., Engtipi, K. and Bala, I. (2019). Magnitude of domestic violence and its socio-demographic correlates among pregnant women in Delhi. *Journal of Family Medicine and Primary Care*, 8 (11), 3634–3639. https://doi.org/10.4103/jfmpc.jfmpc_597_19.

Gleeson, H. (2020) Inside the men's referral service, a call centre dealing with Australia's abusive men and domestic violence. *ABC News*, May 3, 2020. (Accessed May 30, 2020). https://www.abc.net.au/news/2020-05-03/mens-referral-service-family-violence-coronavirus/12207558.

Haag, H. (Lin), Sokoloff, S., MacGregor, N., Broekstra, S., Cullen, N. and Colantonio, A. (2019) Battered and brain injured: Assessing knowledge of traumatic brain injury among intimate partner violence service providers. *Journal of Women's Health*, 28 (7), 990–996.

Heo, M. (2010) Women's movement and the politics of framing: The construction of anti-domestic violence legislation in South Korea, *Women's Studies International*, 33 (3), 225–233.

Hester, M. (2004) Future trends and developments, violence against women in Europe and East Asia. *Violence against Women*, 10 (12), 1431–1448.

Hill, J. (2019) *See What You Made Me Do: Power, Control and Domestic Violence*. Carlton: Schwartz Publishing.

Holland, K.M., Brown, S.V., Hall, J.E. and Logan, J.E. (2018). Circumstances preceding homicide and suicides involving child victims: A qualitative analysis. *Journal of Interpersonal Violence*, 33 (3), 379–401.

Honda, S. and Ogawa, R. (2021) Domestic violence in Japan, an invisible problem in the "safest country in the world". *Deportate, Esuli, Profughe, Rivista Telematica di Studi sulla Memoria Femminile*, 45 (January 2021), 36–59. https://www.unive.it/pag/fileadmin/user_upload/dipartimenti/DSLCC/documenti/DEP/numeri/n45/DEP_45_fileunico.pdf#page=41.

Humphreys, C. and Thiara, R. (2003) Mental health and domestic violence: 'I call it symptoms of abuse'. *British Journal of Social Work*, 33 (2), 209–226.

Hundle, A.K. (2019) Postcolonial patriarchal nativism, domestic violence and transnational feminist research in contemporary Uganda. *Feminist Review*, 121 (1), 37–52.

India Express (2015) 24,771 dowry deaths reported in last 3 years: Govt. *India Express Newspaper*. New Delhi: India Express. Published July 31st. (Accessed March 29, 2017).

Jackman, C. (2020) 'We prefer to pretend this isn't real': The horrific domestic violence threats women face every day. *The New Daily*, April 23, 6:00 am. (Accessed April 23, 2020).

Katz, E. (2019) Coercive control, domestic violence, and a five-factor framework: Five factors that influence closeness, distance, and strain in mother–child relationships. *Violence against Women*, 25 (15). https://journals.sagepub.com/doi/10.1177/1077801218824998.

Kinnersly, P. (2018) New report shows men don't 'just snap'. *Our Watch* Website https://www.ourwatch.org.au/resource/new-report-shows-men-dont-just-snap/.

Klugman, J., Hanmer, L., Twigg, S., Hasan, T., McCleary-Sills, J. and Santa Maria, J. (2014). *Voice and Agency: Empowering Women and Girls for Shared Prosperity*. Washington, DC: World Bank.

Kuan, H. (2021) The law on domestic violence and its practice in Taiwan. *Deportate, Esuli, Profughe, Rivista Telematica di Studi sulla Memoria Femminile*, 45 (January 2021), 25–34.

Kulczycki, A. and Windle, S. (2011). Honor killings in the Middle East and North Africa: A systematic review of the literature. *Violence against Women*, 17 (11), 1442–1464.

Laing, L. (2003) Routine screening for domestic violence in health services. *Australian Domestic and Family Violence Clearinghouse Topic Paper*. Copyright © Australian

Domestic and Family Violence Clearinghouse. https://citeseerx.ist.psu.edu/viewdoc/download?doi=10.1.1.563.2780&rep=rep1&type=pdf.

Laing, L., Irwin, J. and Toivonen, C. (2012) Across the divide: Using research to enhance collaboration between mental health and domestic violence services. *Australian Social Work*, 65 (1), 120–135.

Lansdell, G.T., Saunders, B.J., Eriksson, A., et al. (2022) Strengthening the connection between acquired brain injury (ABI) and family violence: The importance of ongoing monitoring, research and inclusive terminology. *Journal of Family Violence*, 37, 367–380.

Leight, J. (2022) Intimate partner violence against women: A persistent and urgent challenge. *The Lancet (British Edition)*, 399 (10327), 770–771.

Lévesque, S., Rousseau, C. and Dumerchat, M. (2020) Influence of the relational context on reproductive coercion and the associated consequences. *Violence against Women* (Online first). https://journals.sagepub.com/doi/10.1177/1077801220917454.

McQuigg, R.J.A. (2018) Is it time for a UN treaty on violence against women? *The International Journal of Human Rights*, 22 (3), 305–324.

Moulding, N. (2016a) Putting gender in the frame, feminist social work and mental health. In S. Wendt and N. Moulding (eds) *Contemporary Feminisms in Social Work Practice* (1st ed.), 181–195. London: Routledge.

Moulding, N.T. (2016b) *Gendered Violence, Mental Health and Recovery in Everyday Lives: Beyond Trauma*. London: Routledge.

Murphy (2020) Australian government pumps $1bn into health and family violence services as coronavirus spreads. *The Guardian*, Australian Edition, Sunday March 29. (Accessed March 31, 2020). https://www.theguardian.com/australia-news/2020/mar/29/australian-government-to-pump-1bn-into-health-and-family-violence-services-as-coronavirus-spreads.

Murray, S. and Powell, A. (2009) 'What's the problem?' Australian public policy constructions of domestic and family violence. *Violence against Women*, 15 (5), 532–552.

Naghizadeh, S., Mirghafourvand, M. and Mohammadirad, R. (2021). Domestic violence and its relationship with quality of life in pregnant women during the outbreak of COVID-19 disease. *BMC Pregnancy Childbirth*, 21, Article 88. https://link.springer.com/article/10.1186/s12884-021-03579-x.

Namy, S., Carlson, C., O'Hara, K., Nakuti, J., Bukuluki, P., Lwanyaaga, J., Namakula, S., Nanyunja, B., Wainberg, M.L., Naker, D. and Michau, L. (2017). Towards a feminist understanding of intersecting violence against women and children in the family. *Social Science & Medicine (1982)*, 184, 40–48.

Nemeth, J.M., Mengo, C., Kulow, E., Brown, A. and Ramirez, R. (2019) Provider perceptions and domestic violence (DV) survivor experiences of traumatic and anoxic-hypoxic brain injury: Implications for DV advocacy service provision. *Journal of Aggression, Maltreatment & Trauma*, 28 (6), 744–763.

Nikparvar, F., Spencer, C.M. and Stith, S.M. (2021) Risk markers for women's physical intimate partner violence victimization in Iran: A meta-analysis. *Violence against Women*, 27 (11), 1896–1912.

NSWBCSR (NSW Bureau of Crime Statistics and Research) (2016). Incidents of assault (domestic assault) from Oct 2015 to Sep 2016. *NSW Crime Tool*. Sydney: NSW Government. http://crimetool.bocsar.nsw.gov.au/bocsar/.

Oneinthree (2020) One in three men is a victim of domestic violence. https://www.oneinthree.com.au/.

ONS (Office of National Statistics) (2016) Domestic abuse in England and Wales: Year ending March 2016. UK Government. https://www.ons.gov.uk/peoplepopulationandcommunity/crimeandjustice/bulletins/domesticabuseinenglandandwales/yearendingmarch2016.

Orme, J. (2003). It's feminist because I say so!: Feminism, social work and critical practice in the UK. *Qualitative Social Work*, 2, 131–154.

Orpin, J., Papadopoulos, C. and Puthussery, S. (2020) The prevalence of domestic violence among pregnant women in Nigeria: A systematic review. *Trauma, Violence, & Abuse*, 21 (1), 3–15.

Phillips, T. (2022) Mexico: Activists voice anger at Amlo's failure to tackle 'femicide emergency'. *The Guardian*, March 5, 2022. https://www.theguardian.com/world/2020/mar/05/mexico-femicide-emergency-activists.

Prieto-Carrón, M., Thomson, M. and Macdonald, M. (2007) No more killings! Women respond to femicides in Central America. *Gender and Development*, 15 (1), 25–40.

Rice, M. (2001) Japan adopts tough domestic violence law. *Crime and Law*, Women's ENews, December 2, 2001. https://womensenews.org/2001/12/japan-adopts-tough-domestic-violence-law/.

Sardinha, L., Maheu-Giroux, M., Stöckl, H., Meyer, S.R. and García-Moreno, C. (2022) Global, regional, and national prevalence estimates of physical or sexual, or both, intimate partner violence against women in 2018. *The Lancet*, 399 (10327), 803–813.

South Australian Police (2020) Update: Police appeal for information on Morphett Vale murder. April 2020, 1:22 pm. South Australia Police. https://www.police.sa.gov.au/sa-police-news-assets/front-page-news/suspicious-death-at-morphett-vale#.XqvUsZMzY62.

Stark, E. (2007) *Coercive Control: The Entrapment of Women in Personal Life*. New York: Oxford University Press.

Targeted News Service (2020) Global voices: Even with renewed laws, Brazil struggles to protect women amid rising femicide. *Targeted News Service*, March 20, 2020. (Accessed April 13, 2020). https://globalvoices.org/2020/03/19/even-with-renewed-laws-brazil-struggles-to-protect-women-amid-rising-femicide/.

The Economist (2020) Why Latin America treats "femicides" differently from other murders. *The Economist*, March 5, 2020 edition. (Accessed May 2, 2020). https://www.economist.com/the-americas/2020/03/05/why-latin-america-treats-femicides-differently-from-other-murders.

Tsantefski, M., Wilde, T., Young, A. and O'Leary, P. (2018) Inclusivity in interagency responses to domestic violence and child protection. *Australian Social Work*, 71 (2), 202–214.

United Nations (1993). 48/104. Declaration on the elimination of violence against women. http://www.un.org/documents/ga/res/48/a48r104.htm.

UNODC (United Nations Office of Drugs and Crime) (2018) Home, the most dangerous place for women, with majority of female homicide victims worldwide killed by partners or family, UNODC study says. Vienna: UNODC. https://www.unodc.org/unodc/en/press/releases/2018/November/home--the-most-dangerous-place-for-women--with-majority-of-female-homicide-victims-worldwide-killed-by-partners-or-family--unodc-study-says.html.

UN SDGs (2016) Sustainable Development Goals. Geneva: United Nations. (Accessed March 23, 2017). http://www.un.org/sustainabledevelopment/sustainable-development-goals/.

UN Women (2000) The convention on the elimination of all forms of discrimination against women. https://www.un.org/womenwatch/daw/cedaw/.

Villegas, P. (2020) In Mexico, women go on strike nationwide to protest violence. *The New York Times*, March 9, 2020. (Accessed March 15, 2020). https://www.nytimes.com/2020/03/09/world/americas/mexico-women-strike-protest.html.

Wagers, S.M. (2020) Domestic violence growing in wake of coronavirus outbreak. *The Conversation*, April 8, 2020. (Accessed April 9, 2020). https://theconversation.com/domestic-violence-growing-in-wake-of-coronavirus-outbreak-135598.

Weldon, S.L. (2002) *Protest, Policy and the Problem of Violence Against Women, a Cross-National Comparison*. Pittsburgh: University of Pittsburgh Press.

Weldon, S.L. and Htun, M. (2013) Feminist mobilisation and progressive policy change: Why governments take action to combat violence against women. *Gender & Development*, 21 (2), 231–247.

WHO (World Health Organization) (2005) *WHO Multi-country Study on Women's Health and Domestic Violence against Women*. Geneva: WHO. http://www.who.int/gender/violence/who_multicountry_study/summary_report/summary_report_English2.pdf.

WHO (World Health Organization) (2021) Violence against women intimate partner and sexual violence against women. *Fact Sheet* (Updated November 2021). https://www.who.int/news-room/fact-sheets/detail/violence-against-women.

4

FEMINIST PRACTICE, MOTHERHOOD, TRANS PARENTHOOD AND MATERNAL RIGHTS

Introduction

The aim of this chapter is to discuss and illuminate key feminist social welfare practice, activism and social policy issues related to motherhood and maternal rights and welfare for cisgender and queer women and transgender men. As an important part of the feminist agenda since the second wave, motherhood has been central to how women (and, more recently, others not identifying as women and choosing to bear children) are affected by social judgement, religion, morality, medicalisation, market mechanisms, social stigma and legal, economic, welfare and health systems. Bearers and carers of children often have ambiguous social, legal or cultural rights, which if they exist at all, are constantly challenged along with the capacity to have control over their own bodies in child-bearing and caring practices. The social welfare of bearers and carers of children is not only central to the well-being of individuals and families but has been a critical aspect of feminist struggles and debates as it also relates to autonomy over one's body, choice to not have children and to have control over reproductive choice. This chapter focuses on childbirth and the status of and expectations on maternity, motherhood and trans parenthood, whereas the following chapter extends some of these issues in a focus on reproductive control and rights, interventions, welfare and autonomy.

Ideas of motherhood and the social positioning of mothers as a core intersection with other aspects of identity, especially in relation to class or minority status, are also central to this discussion. In many ways, the political and social construction of motherhood is one of the deepest and most entrenched signifiers of sexism and of the persistence of patriarchal views in most societies. This is the case regardless of the advances or success of feminism, the women's movement or ideas and experiences of diverse, non-binary gender identity. bell hooks

DOI: 10.4324/9781315625188-4

commented on this in relation to the then USA President Donald Trump's blatant misogyny:

> And it reinforced a heteronormative vision of decency, not a powerful, passionate argument for justice and for where we stand as people who are advocates of feminist politics. Which is not about whether you're a mom or not, it's about the whole question of whether we can exist without being seen as second-class citizens. This heteronormative vision of parenthood is part of that.
>
> *(Alptraum, 2017)*

In analysing affronts to women's maternal agency, the oppressive consequences of some practices in reproductive and maternal medicine and the impact of social constructions of good or bad mothering, the question of gender inequality arises as an underlying, persistent, unyielding cause. This is not to suggest that women cannot or do not resist the 'traditional' narrative. In fact, feminism has been the central framing of such resistances and evidence of women's collective and individual resistance is plentiful. Within traditional social welfare practice, moral panic about parenting and the protection of children more broadly has a history of, on the one hand, critical intervention to protect children from exploitation and abuse, but on the other hand, deep inroads of moral judgement based on privileged and religious judgement of what children need, resulting in practices of removal of children and persecution of women because of poverty, immorality, addiction, disability or race.

In the last chapter, I focused on feminist responses to how women are subjected to interpersonal violence, in this chapter the focus is on feminist responses to societal and institutional forms of control, violence, social exclusion and oppression related to women's (and transgender men's) unique reproductive capacity and identity. It is noted that reproduction is not commonly considered a core social welfare focus as it has mostly been captured by medicalisation, law and religion, three powerful discourses that often challenge the fundamental agency of women (and transgender men) and their physical status that is intrinsic to their biological sex. However, reproduction and motherhood are central welfare issues related to human rights, sexism, women's poverty and autonomy, the exploitation of women, homophobia and children's welfare and rights.

One area this chapter will not address that should be acknowledged as central to social welfare is 'reproductive labour', which is the essential ongoing parental work of caring for children. Reproductive labour is, as Laura Briggs (2017) points out, the invisible everyday constant care that parents do, is relegated to the private sphere, and rarely acknowledged for its enormous and vital contribution to society and the economy. She also points out how the conservative right of politics in the USA has used reproductive labour in their attacks on feminists and feminism, accusing feminists of only seeing productive labour as rewarding and, in contrast, conservative women are 'pro-family, have husbands and love their children' (Briggs, 2017, pp. 10–21).

Mostly, reproductive labour only gains attention as a welfare issue when parenting has been deemed as *at risk* of failing or is failing, in that it is placing children at risk or causing children harm. It is important to note that feminist concerns about reproductive labour are in parallel to other fissures in gender equality and, as women have traditionally been and are the predominant carers of children, they have advocated strongly for the recognition of reproductive labour as important and equal work for both fathers, mothers and other diverse gender identities who have children. The gains in this sphere are recognisable in countries that have good childcare, universal parental leave, and gender-equal work regulations and pay. However, the benefits from such policies and services are affected by intersecting experiences and identities.

As discussed previously in relation to all feminist concerns, there are significant, intersecting distinctions when considering the extent that women can exercise control over their own reproduction and maternal experiences. This means that in some poorer countries the struggle for rights will be different and often a matter of life or death compared to wealthier countries. Although, as has been noted, there are extreme divergences between people with differing socio-economic statuses within wealthy countries where poverty often excludes many individuals and communities from equal access to rights, services and care. This is particularly exacerbated by intersections of race, religion, ethnicity, class, age, impairment or disability, sexual identity and gender. This chapter will explore feminist understandings of motherhood, mothers' and transgender men's welfare, interventions and practice in relation to maternal health rights, obstetric violence and the loss of a baby.

Transgender Men as Birth Parents

Values and judgements about motherhood or parenthood also impinge on non-binary identified and transgender people's reproductive rights and health. Although this chapter is mostly about women (regardless of their sexual preference) as most people experiencing motherhood and childbirth, much of the key social justice issues are relevant to those who don't identify as women but choose to bear children. As some societies become more accepting and supportive of diverse gender identities, transgender men are increasingly choosing to have children as are others who 'transition' to a legal recognition in the 'preferred gender' resulting in, 'more and more trans people become[ing] parents through sexual intercourse, sperm donation, or assisted reproduction... after legal transitioning' (Margaria, 2020, p. 225). A major legal challenge is the desire for transgender men to be recognised as a father of the child they gave birth to, thus requiring law reform that goes beyond fixed biological identities. One compromised position is to recognise a transgender man as a birth parent and avoid the biological distinction of mother or father (Margaria, 2020). However, given the powerful discourse of motherhood derived from the biological capacity to conceive and give birth to children, there is a tension between a transgender man's identity as a man, his choice to bear a child and his desire to be seen as a father, which fits his gender identity. This not only confronts the heteronormative, conservative structure of family formation, but the everyday health system and services, where his welfare should be supported. Feminist praxis in midwifery and obstetrics is critical to that welfare as it demands equal treatment and recognition of gender identity.

According to reported Australian public health system (Medicare) data, 75 people who identified as male gave birth in 2016 and a further 40 in 2017 (Hattenstone, 2019). Margaria points out, a high level of moral panic has arisen in response to men having babies 'as their visible departure from the conventional imaginary of reproduction that portrays 'male' and 'female' contributions as clearly defined and distinct from one another and, in particular, to the challenges they pose to gendered notions of pregnancy' (2020, p. 225). This kind of societal reaction strengthens the alliance and key commitment of fourth-wave feminism to support transgender people. A global study of 51 research papers on transgender birth and parenthood showed that transgender parents were 'more often subjected to discrimination in contact with authorities' in the context of other (mainly medical) research supporting transgender fertility preservation and calling for increased access to fertility medicine (Gunnarsson Payne and Erbenius, 2018, pp. 331–332). It was also reported that a USA survey on transgender men's experiences of pregnancy and birth confirmed that they often desired to have children and were prepared to become pregnant but raised the problem of accessing 'trans-friendly healthcare providers' (Gunnarsson Payne and Erbenius, 2018, pp. 331–332). There have been significant cultural shifts around transgender men having babies and this has had an impact on their reproductive rights in the process of gender transformations. For example, in Sweden and the UK there had been historical requirements for sterilisation prior to gender reassignment surgeries, which have now changed with the acceptance of transgender men's choice to have a baby (Gunnarsson Payne and Erbenius, 2018, pp. 331–332). The social welfare implications are important for transgender and other non-binary gendered people choosing to be parents. Currently, this issue is only conceivably relevant to some countries in the global North as the many prohibitive views that affect maternity and birth for women are still dominant across the world more generally and create barriers for transgender men.

Motherhood: Impositions and Expectations

The unique status of motherhood in reproduction has been the subject of deep and abiding social expectations, dramatic changes in the status of women, transformations in the roles of women in society, work and the economy, complex and challenging social welfare practices and, of course, its place in feminist thought and action. Motherhood as an unassailable and unique role for women or those who have wombs but don't identify as women, has been celebrated and highly valued as an essential part of human life. However, it is also a status that oppresses, pushes and categorises women into extreme disadvantage both during pregnancy, as a medicalised subject and as a marketable capacity, during parenting and, long after they are no longer carers of young children. The identity of a mother is rarely described without adjectives that indicate whether they are good or bad mothers, or even as failed, barren women for those who can't or do not have children out of choice.

Views of women who choose not to be mothers are highly informed by the deeply patriarchal idea of womanhood as inseparable from motherhood. Apart from denying the agency to choose to be a parent or not, such views often override any context or circumstance or structural limitations to a woman's capacity to be a mother or indeed a 'good mother'. Such mainstream discourses are also exaggerated when applied to non-traditional mothers, women with intellectual or other disabilities, lesbian mothers or transgender parents because the idea of mother comes from such fixed notions of what a mother parent should be like – married, feminine, devoted, womanly, caring, kind, nurturing and selfless. If this is a benchmark for motherhood then, as Nelson and Robertson astutely observe 'what we are seeing is the emergence of a moralizing atmosphere in which all women appear to present a problem' (2018, p. 2) given the highly constraining and oppressive nature of such expectations.

This is a critical point of self-reflexivity for welfare practitioners as, like ageism or racism, deeply entrenched expectations of motherhood become the lens through which mothers, mothers to be, women of a fertile age in general and unconventional mothers are seen and judged. For women in the global North, having a child is fraught with the complexities of the modern world. There is a perpetual swarm of ideas, demands, unsolicited advice, professional resources and the pressure of traditional views of women as being most highly valued because of their capacity to bear children. This includes, of course, the idea of legitimacy that in Judaeo Christian and other religiously underpinned societies means formal legal marriage to the father of a child.

In the contemporary global North's consumerist, neoliberal world an entire market has emerged for what has been termed intensive motherhood (Elliot and Bowen, 2018) where mothers must invest 'quality time' and competitive engagement in the everyday development of their child. In contrast to this are poor mothers who can be viewed as 'withholding, uninformed or neglectful' (Elliot and Bowen, 2018, p. 499). Elliot and Bowen's research with African American mothers in the USA noted that in the age of the intensive mother, 'for mothers of color, gendered racialization put them at particular risk of being labeled as bad mothers… for deviating from expectations' (2018, p. 499). A further impact of neoliberalism on mothering is described by Nelson and Robertson (2018) as the emergence of the 'mumpreneur', where, with the assistance of social media 'at-home mothers' are finding ways of using their children and their mother identity to make money. This is a practice related particularly to girl babies and girls and fashion but also about how the child becomes a social media icon followed by thousands and becomes linked to saleable commodities. Nelson and Robertson make the point, however, that the use of social media celebrity by mothers using their children 'is especially appealing to mothers who feel limited in their social and economic agency' (2018, p. 66). Nelson and Robertson link this phenomenon to the wider expectations of mothers to facilitate their children's material world through consumption. They observed:

> We are living in an age in which emotional and economic relationships have begun to define and shape each other. Economic relationships have become deeply emotional at the same time that our emotional relationships are being redefined through economic language of bargaining and exchange.
>
> *(2018, p. 62)*

From a practice perspective of working with mothers, it is important to be aware of innate judgementalism based on socio-economic class, where mothers might be judged for their excessive consumption of things for their children, then are seen as failing as a parent when they facilitate their child's consumption at the same time that the market it telling them they are failing as a parent if they do not buy specific products or activities for and related to their children (Nelson and Robertson, 2018).

These phenomena are class-based and appear to be an affliction across advanced capitalist societies. In research conducted in Russia, Kuleshova found several differing categories of modern motherhood, including what she described as 'glamour motherhood', where motherhood 'needs to be bright, snazzy, lightweight, optimistic and exclusive' (2015, p. 114). Kuleshova (2015) noted that the babies of such women became super-consumers from the day they were born, thus adding to the notion of the commodification of both motherhood and childhood. This type of motherhood was also detailed as a phenomenon in Australia with the rise of the 'yummy mummy', where being a 'good mother' is related directly through her choices in consumption of goods for herself (ensuring glamour) and her child rather than the act of having children (Goodwin and Huppatz, 2010). Although possibly related to a push-back against traditional notions of the modest, self-sacrificing and selfless mother as part of the success of the freedom to be sexual and sexualised (yummy) that was a cornerstone of third-wave feminism, the rise of the mother who has to look perfect and consume perfectly creates yet another form of social pressure on the contemporary mother, another possible standard that can be failed (Clarke, 2014; Goodwin and Huppatz, 2010). Again, the issue of economic and social class is a big factor in the capacity of mothers to be 'glamorous' and can be seen as a profitable form of marketing and commodification (Clarke, 2010).

Kuleshova's (2015) typologies of motherhood were all linked to the rising influence of [neoliberal] globalisation that feeds divergent views of how to be a mother in Russia today but were distinctive in their factionalism that linked them to differing ideologies such as conforming to religious (orthodox motherhood), business (professional motherhood) feminist (feminist motherhood) and a profusion of ideas via the Internet (cyber motherhood). What was also evident across all 'types', was the absence of the role of fathers and a consistent theme of the burden of motherhood but also the expectations and pressures of the contemporary world on the idea of being a mother.

Of course, the actual material absence of a father (or other partner) that results in sole parenting for a mother creates a different class of motherhood as single mothers (or sole parents) face extreme hardship in any country that does not have a strong welfare support system. The largest group of women in poverty in most country profiles are sole parent mothers. As reported by UN Women:

> The results, presented by Senior Economist of the World Bank, Kinnon Scott, show that between the age of 20 and 34 years, women are more likely to be poor than men. The difference coincides with the peak productive and reproductive ages of men and women and can be related to factors such as having young children in the household and the higher likelihood for women to leave the labour market in response to rising demands on the time they allocate to unpaid care work. Divorce, separation, and widowhood also affect women more negatively than men. Divorced women in the 18–49 age group are more than twice as likely to be poor than divorced men in that same age group.
>
> The research also showed that households with children are among the poorest, and that single parents with children, and predominantly single mothers with children, face a far higher risk of poverty.
>
> *(UN Women, 2017)*

In many contexts, sole-parent mothers are seen as bad mothers, regardless of the reasons why they have taken on being a parent on their own. In Australia, for example, a 'single mother's' pension was introduced in the 1970s, hard fought for by feminists on two major counts, the first being that women had been forced to give up their children into adoption if they were 'unwed' and, second, women needed financial support if they had to leave a violent intimate partner. However, the sole parent pension has undergone several reforms by conservative neoliberal governments, placing conditionalities and expectations of gaining work in the labour force once their youngest child reaches school age. Such policy shifts are to ensure that sole parent mothers cannot *choose* to be an at-home (good) mother (as they might in a normative two-parent family) asserting the view that a sole parent without a spouse must become the breadwinner (a non-traditional, bad mother) – responsible for the economic status of their children.

From a feminist practice point of view, this means that the struggle to 'liberate' women from often oppressive, normative notions of a good and 'proper' mother requires advocacy for change across market, political, legal, social, religious, welfare, health and community battle lines. Dominant neoliberal thinking has contributed to a further pressure on mothers by justifying the reduction of direct transfers in welfare support through the ideological goal towards less state, particularly less welfare state. The impact of this trend in countries such as

Australia and the UK has been seen in the rise of conditionality for mothers on welfare and has resulted in a dramatic increase in homeless sole parent mothers and greater stress and stigmatisation (BBC News, 2018; Manne, 2018; Phillips, 2017; Syal, 2019).

Motherhood Rights

Like many social issues that are highly divergent based on economic and social class, extreme differences in the experiences of motherhood are not only obvious in relation to what the state does or does not offer and what women can afford in rich or poor countries. We have also seen the emergence of contemporary exploitation of motherhood by the global North of the global South. This has occurred in multiple ways through history, with the theft of children into servitude and adoption, through to international adoptions sanctioned between sovereign states and to the more recent technologically assisted exploitations/market exchanges through surrogate mothers. As the countries of those seeking to exploit healthy wombs for surrogacy are often countries that have had past colonial ties with the poorer countries, this can be seen as a manifestation of neo-colonialism, embodied in the body of the surrogate mother.

Historically, domestic adoptions and contemporary international adoptions are inextricably bound up with 'poor mother' judgments related to poverty or 'neglect' and what a more wealthy or 'stable' family can provide a child. Social welfare is on both sides of this equation as social workers, medical staff, politicians, and lawyers have sought to both facilitate, punish and exploit vulnerable mothers as well as what they see as acting in the best interests of children. Feminist activists in welfare made significant inroads into protecting mothers' rights in relation to adoption from the early 1970s onwards in the global North, asserting the need for income support and legal protections for single mothers. This was while the women's movement fought for and gained reproductive rights to contraception and legal abortion, thus reducing the overall number of young single mothers in many global North countries. This was a far more successful achievement in secular and rich countries than it was in heavily religious cultures and poorer countries. The rights of mothers, regardless of their marital status, to keep previously defined 'unwanted' children created a push for new sources of babies for infertile couples and international adoptions grew rapidly.

A further instance of institutional imposition on 'bad' mothers is exemplified by the experience of mothers who become prisoners. Data from Australia indicates that there has been a significant increase in women prisoners and that 85 per cent of women going to prison had been pregnant at some time in their lives, one in two were mothers, 2 per cent were pregnant, a third were Indigenous women and 50 per cent had a history of mental illness (AIHW, 2019). Regardless of how they came to prison mothers generally want to be with their children and do not want their children to end up in foster care as so many had been fostered in their childhoods (Walker et al., 2019). For women who are mothers of babies or very young children in Australian prisons the conditions are not conducive to parenting and their motherhood is under surveillance constantly by prison guards who judge their parenting skills and can breach them, which results in their children being removed (Walker et al., 2019).

Escude and Law (2013) examined the status of incarcerated mothers across several countries in the Americas where feminist interventions supported calls for the rights of mothers to have proper care for children where they were allowed to keep their very young children with them in prison or to institute reforms that allowed for mothers to undergo home arrest up until their children reached the age of five years as was the case for some women in Argentina. However, in the USA they noted that 147,000 children's mothers had their parental rights terminated when they entered prison and that in 2007, over 65,000 women in state and federal prisons were mothers to minor children and largely primary carers before being arrested (Escude and Law, 2013). They also found that 'children of incarcerated mothers are five times more likely to be placed in foster care than children of incarcerated fathers' and a law passed in 1997, the federal Adoption and Safe Families Act (ASFA), required the cessation of parents' legal rights if a child was in foster care for 15 out of 22 months (Escude and Law, 2013, p. 13). Such children were then placed in permanent adoption.

However, feminist welfare interventions did occur in some prisons and groups. Such an example was the New York State-based Women's Prison Association and the Volunteers of Legal Services, which created an advocacy group, the Incarcerated Mother's Law group that sought to assist incarcerated mothers with their rights as mothers in the prison system (Escude and Law, 2013, p. 14). As noted by other researchers the ASFA had a greater impact on African American families as it was applied extensively beyond the prison system in child protection cases of poverty, neglect, and drug addiction (Curtis and Denby, 2004). This is a form of systemic prejudice against mothers that is deeply based in issues of race and poverty and is not unlike the historical legacy of colonised states and Indigenous populations.

In Australia, there had been a long history of the removal (commonly understood as theft) of lighter-skinned Aboriginal children from their mothers to 'rescue' them from their identities as Aboriginal and the poverty and exclusion that were imposed on Aboriginal communities through colonisation, dispossession, displacement and state control (Fejo-King, 2011; Tedmanson and Fejo-King, 2016). The extreme injustices imposed by state-sanctioned notions of correct motherhood extended to all Indigenous families because of the lack of recognition of culture and due to poverty arising from social exclusion that was then deemed to be neglect. For many Indigenous women, such impositions continue today as Indigenous families experience a disproportionate number of child removals by welfare authorities at seven times the rate of non-Indigenous children (Evershed and Allam, 2018; Fejo-King, 2011) and have conditions placed on their income support to force compliance to 'good mothering' through income quarantining (Bielefeld, 2012).

The impact of the 'Stolen Generation' of children has deeply hurt all Indigenous communities in Australia and after a National Inquiry into its history and deeply felt effects, some fostering arrangements became more sensitive to Indigenous needs, culture and identity, and extended families were recognised as the key carers of children who could not be cared for by parents (Bringing Them Home Report, 1997). However, Indigenous families had fought for changes long before the inquiry, and in some states, the system of fostering had already been recognised as a process that had to be in the hands of local Indigenous communities. Although, as noted above, this has not resulted in a resolved or satisfactory system of care and the social problems that are intrinsic to judgements of neglect and abuse, namely drug and alcohol addiction, unemployment and poverty remain. This is largely due to the long-term impact of colonisation and ongoing racism and social exclusion as well as European cultural views of motherhood. Despite the obvious failure to support the status of Indigenous parenting in Australia and other similar settler nations, increased awareness of white policymakers and administrations about the destructive impositions of colonisation on Indigenous populations has led to greater understanding of the importance of culture and identity. Consequently, some programs and activist groups have evolved in postcolonial states to redress the historical theft of children from their mothers through support for self-determination.

In this respect, many countries have reformed their laws to recognise Indigenous rights in relation to their children, and through widespread availability of contraception and social support for sole parent mothers, the global North has exported its 'market' for adoptable children for infertile people who want children. This has occurred in a range of ways, including inter-country adoption. Inter-country adoption is a complex process that has seen constant negotiation and re-negotiation between states, depending often on internal policies and economic context and in many cases, it has been a way of saving children from a harsh life of institutional care. However, there are adoption processes that are not mediated by states effectively and exploitation of mothers does occur.

In an in-depth study by Claudia Fonseca in relation to the Brazilian Favelas, she made the following observation of relinquishing mothers caught up in a class-based international adoption program with the USA:

> In the Brazilian case I examine here, ...not only were the birth mothers I dealt with ill-versed in their own individual rights, but also their heterogeneous racial backgrounds (African, Native American, Polish, Portuguese) provided them with no evident common identity through which to articulate their resistance.
>
> Indeed, these women were seen, and, in general, saw themselves as nothing other than "poor" - raising doubts in many people as to whether they had any "culture" at all.

(2002, p. 400)

Here Fonseca (2002) is referring to the fact that in postcolonial states where first peoples have experienced the theft of their children, as part of the action of colonisation, they have, in recent history, be able to utilise their culture as resistance and argue for children to be adopted into their own communities, as had been a traditional practice for centuries amongst many groups of people, Indigenous Australians, Aboriginal Canadians and Native Americans for example (Fonseca, 2002, p. 399). Feminists have been divided on the issue of adoption, but many feminist social workers and advocates have worked closely with mothers and families to support them staying together with their children and have identified the process of adoption, in many cases, as an infringement on a mother's human rights and often the children of adoption have also joined this position as they have discovered the lack of choice their mothers had in 'giving them up'.

Feminist activists engaged in social welfare have faced difficult challenges in working with mothers who are judged as bad mothers due to the perceived 'risks' their actions place on their children. Adoption is one area but another issue for this struggle is child labour in poor economies. For example, Leigh Campoamor (2016) conducted a study with poor mothers who required their children to work in the informal economy to assist with the family income and developed an understanding of this process that led to the idea of 'defensive motherhood'. Campoamor found that rather than exercising exploitation, the mothers whose children worked performing or selling goods on the streets in Lima, Peru, were motivated by the need to maintain safe housing and keeping their children in education and that their perceived 'bad motherhood' was due to a failure by the state, and others judging them, to recognise the 'structural oppression, economic injustice and cultural traditions' that motivated this form of child labour (2016, p. 153). As she further observed, 'narratives of responsibility linked to the idea of the exploitative mother deflect attention away from the varied meanings and motives that children and their families attach to work, reinforcing structural violence of poverty and inequality' (Campoamor, 2016, p. 154). This example points to the importance of advocacy for mothers experiencing poverty and demands for appropriate state support through an inclusive, strong welfare state.

Maternal Death and Abuse

Maternal death occurs for different reasons, but it most commonly occurs due to poor health and poor care during pregnancy and during childbirth. This is a highly gendered issue and is an important aspect of women's (and transgender men who choose to give birth) welfare across the world. Although high rates of maternal mortality usually occur in the global South, the case of African American women in the USA suggests intersectionality is a significant factor at times of increased vulnerability. African American women in the USA have been dying at three times the rate of white women in the 21st century. A five-year average of national data in the USA from 2011 to 2015 estimated a mortality rate at

20.7 per cent for every 100,000 live births (Ollove, 2018). This rate placed it alongside countries that have extensive poverty and political and/or economic instability – such as Afghanistan, Lesotho and Swaziland, all countries with rising rates of maternal morbidity (Ollove, 2018). According to the Center for Disease Control and Prevention (2018) during 2011–2014, there were 12.4 deaths per 100,000 live births for white women compared to 40 deaths per 100,000 live births for black women. In the state of New Jersey, the maternal death rate for Black women was seven times than that of white women in 2021 (Governor Phil Murphy, 2021).

This growth in very poor maternal mortality rates for African American women occurred during a period when interventions driven by the United Nations Millennium Development Goals, saw a 43 per cent decrease in maternal mortality worldwide (UNFPA, 2017). The causes of high maternal mortality are consistent in most geographical locations: poverty; distance from medical care; lack of information; inadequate services; cultural practices; untreated chronic conditions and a lack of access to health care, especially in rural areas where hospitals and maternity units have closed in the past few years due to austerity measures (Ollove, 2018; UNFPA, 2017; WHO, 2018). Improvements came about through advances as simple as recognising that economic inequality was a major factor in appropriate antenatal care and access to a minimum of four visits to a doctor during pregnancy, as was strategically addressed in several global South countries (UNFPA, 2017). For example, Cambodia lifted access for women in the lowest economic status group from less than 25 per cent attending antenatal care to above 50 per cent, thus decreasing maternal deaths significantly (UNFPA, 2017, p. 28). This suggests that getting antenatal care is important but based on the USA's increases in maternal death, especially for African American women, there is a far more complex interrelationship between gender, poverty and race and medical treatment. One of the reasons for higher rates of maternal death for African American women was that they were not listened to by medical staff (Center for Disease Control and Prevention, 2018). Feminist practice in this field would seek to ensure that not only do women have appropriate information about the value of ante or prenatal care but would be facilitated to use services that sought to overcome issues like not being listened to by developing a women-centred service.

Reporting in the New York Times on the alarming rate of maternal deaths in the USA, Kim Brooks (2018) relayed Thea's personal account of her treatment:

> The doctor informed Thea that she'd need to be induced right away. Thea questioned this directive, asking about the success rates for induction and whether she should consider a caesarean section instead. The doctor said she had no choice. She then asked if she could go home to get her overnight bag. She was told, she said, that if she left she could be "arrested for endangering the life of a child."… she remembers this confrontation with her doctor as the moment it became clear to her that in becoming a mother,

she was no longer seen as a person: "I really felt like I was a piece of meat, like I was not being considered in this. It was all about the baby."

(Brooks, 2018)

Brooks (2018) also reported that Alabama voters had recently approved a constitutional amendment recognising 'foetal personhood', a legal tool to 'further curtail the rights of pregnant women in favour of the safety of' a foetus. This is based on the same deeply patriarchal notion that women as mothers have no agency of their own. Instead, the child is more important therefore the choice is taken from the mother, she has no rights of self-determination.

In efforts to address the continued high rate of maternal deaths in the USA, efforts were made to explore why women were dying in childbirth in the richest nation on earth, but 30 out of the 50 states did not attempt to do this. Instead, the women victims were blamed for their own deaths (Brooks, 2018).

>...many state committees emphasized lifestyle choices and societal ills in their reports on maternal deaths. They weighed in on women smoking too much or getting too fat or on their failure to seek prenatal medical care. Mothers, it seems, in addition to being held solely responsible for every facet of their child's well-being, are also being held responsible for their own deaths.
>
> *(Brooks 2018)*

The state of California has been an exception in the USA and

>has made a difference in part by focusing narrowly on problems that arise during labour and delivery, using data collection to quickly identify deficiencies (such as failing to have the right supplies on hand or performing unnecessary Caesarean sections) and training nurses and doctors to overcome them.
>
> *(Ollove, 2018)*

The Californian state Department of Public Health reported that it lowered its maternal mortality rate by 55 per cent, from a high of 16.9 down to 7.3 deaths for every 100,000 live births between 2006 and 2013 (Ollove, 2018).

In another context, Indigenous Canadian feminist activist, Minu Tulugak, was part of a community movement to address birthing rights for her community in Puvirnituq, a small village in Nunavik in the northern region of Quebec, Canada. In resistance to Canadian government policy that required women to travel vast distances away from their community to give birth, in 1985 they organised a movement that would train Indigenous midwives and create a birthing centre for Indigenous women, the Inuulitsivik Maternity (Coast et al., 2016). The key motivation was to ensure that women remained in their community and were supported in traditional community ways in giving birth (Payne, 2010). In another similar community, Inukjuak, the movement has proved very successful, following the same model. Overall, this dramatic shift in local community-based birthing and support had resulted in very low morbidity rates compared to the rest of the nation and a very low caesarean rate for births (Douglas, 2006).

Even though there is little comparison with the high rates of maternal mortality rate (MMR) in the USA, as Australia, with its universal healthcare system, has one of the lowest rates in the world (8.5 deaths per 100,000 live births), there is still a large disparity between Indigenous and non-Indigenous Australian women. According to the Australian government's Institute of Health and Welfare (2017), Aboriginal and Torres Strait Islander women were significantly more likely to die in association with pregnancy and childbirth than other Australian women although the difference was decreasing. Data showed that in

> 1991–1993 the MMR for Aboriginal and Torres Strait Islander women was 4 times that of other Australian women (23.3 per 100,000 women giving birth versus 5.8 per 100,000 women giving birth). In 2012–2014 the MMR for Aboriginal and Torres Strait Islander women was 2.4 times that of other Australian women (13.3 per 100,000 women giving birth versus 5.6 per 100,000 women giving birth).
>
> *(AIHW, 2017)*

The period of the steady decline reflects the development and strengthening of the universal health care system and greater self-determination for Indigenous women's health over that time. However, the ongoing disparity reflects the kind of institutional and resource discrimination that occurs with the intersection of race and poverty.

Feminist practice as social justice practice in relation to Australia's First Nation Peoples requires deep listening to the specific cultural and diverse geographical needs of practices around childbirth. Knowledge about traditional community practices is important, and should be part of a socially justice support system for women from traditional and urban communities:

> …in most traditional groups the elder women decide who will best support a particular woman as she gives birth -- after all, she may not get on too well with her sister-in-law, aunty or whoever, or perhaps there is no relation of the designated kin, and an appropriate alternative will have to be chosen. Certainly, the guiding rule is for the birthing woman to be accompanied by those who will make her feel totally at ease and loved throughout the birthing process… Ngaanyatjarra [lands are in the central Eastern part of Western Australia] women, like the Benin women in Africa, may give birth on their own, away from the rest of their clan. In a broader sense of reality, they do not experience the confusion, isolation or fear that often accompanies the modern experience of birthing in a room full of strangers…
>
> *(Rawlings, 1998)*

It is also important to recognise that in Australia, as in the USA in its bias of greater deaths for African American women, the actual cause of maternal deaths is directly connected to lower quality access to antenatal care and general health care and poverty, which in turn is related to racially based assumptions and exclusion from that which is available through white privilege, as well as long-lasting historical impositions. Colonisation and slavery have deeply affected the social and economic place and status of people of colour and Indigenous peoples and must be acknowledged and understood for successful feminist welfare practice.

Obstetric Violence

For feminists working in any capacity with women entering the health system for childbirth, it is important to consider the risks and occurrences of institutional, gendered violence that can occur at a time of extreme vulnerability. The incidence of imposed procedures is one aspect of this but also the nature of hospitalisation and visceral bullying that occurs against women in childbirth that has both a history of patriarchal domination and, more recently, technological, and institutional violence. The excessive medicalisation of childbirth has seen it become a commodified and marketised process that is often tested based on efficiency within the medical system. These are forms of obstetric violence.

In 2007, a law was passed in Venezuela that included a definition of obstetric violence as:

> (1) Untimely and ineffective attention of obstetric emergencies; (2) Forcing the woman to give birth in a supine position, with legs raised, when the necessary means to perform a vertical delivery are available; (3) Impeding the early attachment of the child with his/her mother without a medical cause thus preventing the early attachment and blocking the possibility of holding, nursing or breast-feeding immediately after birth; (4) Altering the natural process of low-risk delivery by using acceleration techniques, without obtaining voluntary, expressed and informed consent of the woman; (5) Performing delivery via caesarean section, when natural childbirth is possible, without obtaining voluntary, expressed, and informed consent from the woman.
>
> *(D'Gregorio, 2010. p. 201)*

Argentina, Mexico, Chile and Brazil also have laws in place to eliminate obstetric violence however there is little evidence of it being acknowledged in the rest of the world. As noted by the international NGO, *Make Mothers Matter*, it is almost impossible for women to report obstetric violence, given the normalisation of medical and institutional practices and little capacity for legal protection or action (MMM, 2017).

Global research, completed in 2015, gathered data from 169 countries that included 98·4 per cent of the world's births, and estimated that 29.7 million births occurred through caesarean section, 'which was almost double the number of births by this method in 2000' (Boerma et al., 2019). The research showed a link with a major surge in countries where there was a greater use of health centres involved in birthing, particularly in the Latin American and Caribbean region (Boerma et al., 2019). According to extensive international research, this is an indicator of worse outcomes for many women as 'Caesarean delivery continues to result in increased maternal mortality, maternal and infant morbidity, and increased complications for subsequent deliveries, as well as increased financial costs' (OECD, 2019). Given that many of the countries with very high caesarean delivery are in the global South or have large groups of marginalised Indigenous or other minority populations, these statistics raise serious questions about how appropriate this medical intervention in childbirth is. The research also indicates that some caesarean deliveries may not be medically required. According to Brazil's Ministry of Health (Ministério da Saúde) in 2015, 40 per cent of deliveries in the public health system were by caesarean section (Gil, 2017). In Turkey in 2016, it was a rate of over 50 per cent of live births, compared to other countries such as Norway (16 per cent), France (21 per cent), or New Zealand (24 per cent) (OECD, 2019).

Highlighting continued, widespread obstetric violence, there have been increasing reports of systematic caesarean sections as a means of processing women giving birth through the health system as a form of efficiency in several South American countries (Gil, 2017). Also, in Mexico and Bolivia, routine sterilisation or insertion of inter-uterine devices without a woman's consent has occurred (Dixon, 2015; IJRC, 2017). Further, in Mexico, obstetricians have boasted about their invasive techniques of manually and chemically speeding up labour due to:

> ...clinicians' stressful work environment and class-based stereotypes of low-income women results in the routinizing of inhumane medical practices. Hospital overcrowding due to health reforms means that clinicians have to move women swiftly through the system....it also manifests in micro-practices of clinicians that become so routinized that they ultimately have little medical use.
>
> *(Smith-Oka, 2013, p. 597)*

These are also acts of obstetric violence. The WHO noted that unnecessary 'caesarean sections can increase the risk of maternal morbidity, neonatal death and neonatal admission to an intensive care unit' and concerns are also raised 'that in low-income countries in general and among the poorer sections of the populations in such countries in particular – caesarean sections are not always accessible, even when they are clearly indicated' (WHO, 2013). This suggests that it is an overused medical intervention in some countries and an underused medical assistance in others where it may be necessary to save the mother. In both cases, women lose out to forms of rationalisation of resources and lose their agency at a fundamentally important time in motherhood. In China, there has been a dramatic drop in the number of caesarean sections, data showed that in relation to seven million births in 438 hospitals the rate went from 67 per cent of births as caesarean section to 49 per cent in 2016 (Owen and Razak, 2019). However, this dramatic decrease was brought about through the authoritarian government introducing punitive measures against hospitals if they did not show dramatic reductions in the number of caesarean sections performed (Owen and Razak, 2019). Although on the one hand, this sounds like a success story; on the other hand, it has meant that women who need caesarean sections for health reasons may not have them, especially poor rural women. This tension between imposing an unnecessary procedure to many women, to denying a life and death procedure to those who require it demonstrates how important individually tailored support is required, which overcomes economic, social, and geographical disadvantage, in other words, a woman-centred approach.

In one study of obstetric practices in Mexico, it was found that Mexican midwives had created a movement against obstetric violence via a concerted campaign for legislation and through systematic training of future midwives as feminist practitioners acting in the interests of women during childbirth (Dixon, 2015). This was a campaign based on feminist practice and feminist analysis of existing forms of obstetric violence. Dixon (2015) observed:

> …as midwives reflect on the violence they observe within hospitals…what they are trying to articulate is that structural violence *is* physical violence; a common phrase linked to the movement argues that *violencia obstétrica es violencia de genero* – obstetric violence is gendered violence.
>
> *(2015, p. 438)*

Dixon noted that this was a distinctive movement compared to previous feminist analyses that sought to humanise obstetric practices (making them more pleasant and homely), as the Mexican midwives theorised their challenges as feminists and sought to bring attention to the medicalisation of childbirth 'in a way that reflects particular constellations of gender, power and history of biomedicine in Mexico today' (2015, p. 438). In Dixon's interviews with student midwives, it was evident that they were seeing the practices through a feminist lens and were developing sites of resistance. For example, against the common practice of obstetricians inserting contraceptive devices into women immediately after childbirth *without their consent* or knowledge – noting that the obstetricians didn't want poor women having any more babies (Dixon, 2015, p. 441). This is an excellent example of feminist practice. The strategic goals of the midwives were to ensure that through bringing about transformations in the education of future midwives, structural change would occur through future feminist practices and a changed narrative of what childbirth in medical centres should be like.

In response to the United Nations Millennium Development Goals a widespread program, Janani Suraksha Yojana (meaning safe motherhood scheme), was implemented in India to address the very high maternal and natal mortality rates

(Khan et al., 2010). This scheme was launched in all states of India in 2005 and was a direct cash transfer scheme to get women into a medicalised birth setting (Chaturvedi et al., 2015). The main objective of the program was to motivate mainly rural women into at least attending antenatal check-ups and bringing them into an institutional delivery context, as well as some postnatal follow-up (Khan et al., 2010). It has been reported as a highly effective program in achieving those aims but the actual experience for the women moving into an institutional setting has been less positive. Several different studies of the program found extensive obstetric violence in health/birth centres. For example:

> Three themes emerged from the data: 1) the delivery environment is chaotic: delivery rooms were not conducive to safe, women-friendly care provision, and coordination between providers was poor. 2) Staff do not provide skilled care routinely: this emerged from observations that monitoring was limited to assessment of cervical dilatation, lack of readiness to provide key elements of care, and the execution of harmful/unnecessary practices coupled with poor techniques. 3) Dominant staff, passive recipients: staff sometimes threatened, abused, or ignored women during delivery; women were passive and accepted dominance and disrespect. Attendants served as 'go-betweens' patients and providers.
>
> *(Chaturvedi et al., 2015, p. 1)*

Chaturvedi's (2015) research reported that women were being slapped for making a noise during labour, being denied the company of family, and feeling isolated and unsupported in general. In the global North, there are also examples of how the medical establishment passes judgement about women seeking greater agency in the birthing process. Linda Rawlings, a woman who had previously given birth to two babies at home, described her experience:

> My "due date" came and went. During the last three weeks of my pregnancy, I came in contact with numerous health professionals at all levels of the hospital hierarchy. It seemed everyone was eager to get my baby out one way or another. My husband and I preferred to wait. In the course of my dialogue with practitioners I was told that my uterus "would explode," that I was lucky to have given birth to two children without ever having an internal examination "because there are disasters here every day as a result of that." I was told: "if you were my private patient, you'd be in surgery right away whether you liked it or not." When I asked to postpone the possibility of a caesarean until after the weekend (because elective sections aren't performed on Saturday or Sundays), I was quizzed as to "whether the stars would be in a better position then?" I was also asked what I would do if the hospital wouldn't let me come back after the weekend and warned that if I had to have an emergency caesarean, I "might end up with a

hysterectomy, but by then you will have passed out, and we will be saving your life, so you might as well sign the consent form now".

(Rawlings, 1998)

This narrative of judgement demonstrates the continued imposition of power that denies a woman's sense of her own capacity and agency, drawing on lived experience and earned wisdom to make decisions about their own body. This discourse works against women, not with women.

Several studies in countries that continue to have strong patriarchal social structures including Ghana, Kenya, Ethiopia, Nepal and Melawi, have shown men's reluctance to be involved with their wife or partner's maternal experience, including childbirth, results in poorer outcomes for women (Atuahene et al., 2017). Research has also shown that when a man is actively involved, women are more likely to get proper antenatal and maternal healthcare and give birth in a medically supported facility thus reducing maternal and natal mortality rates (Atuahene et al., 2017). Although this implies that it is due to the recognition of greater authority residing with men, fathers, in these diverse cultural contexts, feminist practice, as midwives, social workers, other health professionals and family counsellors, encourages men's participation in the entire parenting process to share the responsibility and work and ensure appropriate support for women's reproductive health and labour.

In the wider sphere of maternity and birth, feminist practice is strongly reflected in the global network of midwives and is highly women centred (Anolack, 2015; Leap, 2009). Laws and debates related to foetal personhood can be seen as disengaging women's autonomy from their motherhood, as the needs of an unborn baby may be prioritised over the needs and wishes of a mother. The antithesis of forms of institutional abuse for women giving birth is the right of women to choose where and how they give birth. In a report on homebirth as a choice Mimi Niles (midwife and PhD candidate at the NYU Rory Meyers College of Nursing) was quoted in pointing out how often the entire well-being of a woman is excluded from the 'birth conversation':

> If we continue to unilaterally focus on safety and risk management, we fail to see the deeper personal, moral, and ethical choices that are often at the center of a person choosing to labor outside of a historically restrictive and paternalistic medical system… Safety is more than just leaving the hospital with an infant in arms, "Niles says." It is also about the mental, emotional and spiritual safety that a new parent needs to transition into the heavy lift of parenting.

> (Hosseine, 2019)

Niles also made the point that due to the very high incidents of maternal mortality amongst African American women, who report being ignored and terrified in hospital settings, they are choosing home births as a way of preserving 'their control and agency' (Hosseine, 2019). Further to that, there is a growing movement in the global North toward 'free birthing', where potential parents opt for a no medical attention or intervention birth (Jackson et al., 2020). In a study of Australian women choosing this birthing practice, Jackson et al. (2020) reported that many of the women choosing this path did it because they had had negative hospital experiences. They reported that globally, between 20 and 48 per cent of women reported having had traumatic birth experiences (Jackson et al., 2020). They observed the study participants:

> Similarly, the majority of the participants in this study perceived their previous birth experiences to be emotionally, mentally, socially, culturally and physically unsafe and as a result, traumatizing. For these women, the choice to *birth outside the system* came from a desire to prevent a repeat of past traumatic events.
>
> *(Jackson et al.)*

Like the findings in Hosseine's (2019) research, this study pointed to a lack of support, poor communication and non-consensual procedures, such as being held down for vaginal examinations (Jackson et al., 2020). Given the intense impact of the Covid-19 pandemic on hospital systems, and the very restrictive impact it had on women attending hospitals to give birth, research was conducted by the King's College London that surveyed 1,754 women who were either pregnant or had given birth since the beginning of pandemic lockdowns (Summers, 2020). They found of the 1,418 pregnant women (still pregnant in April 2020), one in 20 were considering a freebirth with only one who planned it prior to the pandemic, an exceptionally high number compared to the usual number of home births in England and Wales (Summers, 2020). Even though the risk of Covid infection was one reason for this trend, many of the women cited poor previous experiences of childbirth in the hospital setting and saw the choice of only being assisted by a doula (a non-medically trained birth attendant) was an empowering, autonomous choice free of the abuses they had previously experienced in the medical system (Summers, 2020). The extent of obstetric abuse, across the world, is high despite the efforts of feminist practitioners in hospital settings. The essential failures of the system appear to be part of a tendency to control and in some cases abuse women's bodies. It is clearly still a frontline of feminist struggle for women's birthing autonomy, appropriate medical care, and social and emotional support in both the global North and the global South.

Losing a Baby

A further example of the problem of medicalisation of childbirth, but not deeply addressed by feminist researchers and practitioners, usually takes place in the hospital system or at home when a child is stillborn. In many cases, practices related to the death of a newborn baby have improved in the Global North, now treated with high levels of sensitivity and recognition of loss and grief, driven by women-centred midwives who will ensure that the baby is held and recognised as a child by the mother or parents and a birth certificate is issued (Cacciatore and Wieber Lens, 2019). In the past, women were placed in an unconscious state and their baby was whisked away before they could see or touch their child. The transformation of treatment of the stillborn has occurred because practices evolved that recognise parent's attachment to a baby prior to birth but also a woman's right to be recognised as a mother of a child. However, it is estimated that there are 2.6 million stillbirths annually across the world, and 98 per cent happen in low and middle-income countries (Gopichandran et al., 2018). It is also estimated that more than half of stillborn babies are due to preventable causes. In one study in India, it was found that women who experienced stillbirths felt high levels of grief and guilt and described an 'insensitive health system, health care providers, friends, and neighbours', 'poor quality of services provided in the health system and reported that the health care providers were inconsiderate and insensitive' (Gopichandran et al., 2018, p. 1). They felt judged and accused of failing in their motherhood.

In the global North, a woman would most likely know before-hand that her baby had died because there would be a medical check-up and an ultra-sound (although many deaths do occur during childbirth) (Cacciatore and Wieber Lens, 2019) that would mean she would at least avoid the sudden shock experienced by the Indian women interviewed in the above-mentioned study who faced the actual birth process not knowing. It appears that there is still a range of social constraints on acknowledging the loss of a baby at birth in the global North and the global South, views that it is not as bad a losing a child, the failure to publicly acknowledge the loss and the assumption that mothers will recover quickly. Feminists in the 1970s created support groups for women who had experienced stillbirths, recognising the need for support and acknowledgement of their grief (Cacciatore and Wieber Lens, 2019). The importance of public acknowledgement of loss and grief must be recognised, including in medical responses. As pointed out by Cacciatore and Wieber Lens (2019), it is important that people involved in the welfare and health of mothers losing a baby are strong advocates of proper recognition of the grief and loss that women (and men and fathers) experience through a range of sensitive practices at the time of loss of the baby, but also recommended that mothers be made aware of what could happen:

> Another important step to empower women is to inform mothers of the chance of stillbirth... Proper warnings of the risk will better enable mothers to monitor their own babies, especially near the end of their pregnancies. The risk of stillbirth is low, but the consequence is ultimate, and mothers need to know.
>
> *(2019, p. 316)*

It is also important to note that the mother's focus in traditional birthing settings where there is a loss of a baby can fail to sufficiently account for feelings of loss and grief that fathers feel (Riggs et al., 2018). It is important in feminist practice to recognise the experience of loss is equal for a father or same-sex partner, in most cases and support for their feelings must be part of welfare practice in the event of the loss of a baby.

Although the complexities discussed above have been presented as they relate to cis-gender women, they are very similar to transgender or non-binary men who lose babies through miscarriage or still birth. In an international qualitative study of transgender men, non-binary people and men's experiences of pregnancy loss it was found that there had been limited prior research and that there was a need to document the specific issues that the people in their study encountered, particularly in the health system (Riggs et al., 2018). Areas of practice that required particular attention regarding the welfare of transgender men, non-binary people, and men were experiences of clinical service provision following pregnancy loss, the need for formal and informal ongoing support and acknowledging the range of feelings, including grief and loss, 'in order to ensure that experiences of pregnancy loss are acknowledged and heard' (Riggs et al., 2018). The attention to equal treatment includes issues such as the capacity to recognise gender identity in the record keeping and institutional care by addressing the assumption that only women have babies and 'ensuring that medical experiences following a pregnancy loss do not further compound the potential grief experienced by men, trans/masculine, and non-binary people, and their partners' (Riggs et al., 2018).

Still birth or miscarriage are not the only ways a baby can be lost at birth. For decades children have been removed from women at birth based on medicalised, criminal justice and societal judgements about their fitness to parent. Feminist social workers and midwives have been at the forefront of arguing for a more mother-centred perspective in cases of child protection that lead to child removal. Removal of a baby from a mother immediately after childbirth is an area where the feminist practice has had to battle core gendered institutional practices and assumptions. More broadly in child protection interventions, a critical feminist lens is important to achieve a social justice approach. Dunkerley (2017) summarised five feminist principles (drawn from earlier scholars) for feminist practice in this context. They included: 'rejecting false dichotomies' whilst considering the 'inter-relatedness of person and environment', reconceptualising power relations, understanding how a process affects an outcome, the 'value in renaming' and the 'personal is political' (Dunkerley, 2017, p. 252). As discussed earlier in this chapter, the good mother bad mother juxtaposition is a false dichotomy referred to in Dunkerley's (2017) first principle, 'bad mothers' are seen to fail to always place their child's welfare above their own and can be perceived as bad due to existing prejudices base on intersections of poverty, addiction, living in a violent relationship, having a disability or having a racial identity that is seen to suggest parenting risks. As Dunkerley (2017) further notes, the focus on child welfare can often fail to account for a mother's complex relationship and social and economic environment.

Most governments have statutes that seek to protect children from harm. Social workers are most commonly given the statutory responsibility to decide if a child faces too great a risk to go home with their mother. This is generally based on a history of child protection issues, such as a context of domestic violence, a judgement about whether a disability affects capacity to parent, a history of drug addiction and so on. Social workers with this responsibility are acting in the interests of the child but usually have a lot of knowledge of the family dynamics and the individual experiences of the mother or parents of such a child. Social workers often advocate for keeping a child with their mother and are often active in parenting support that aims to do so. Social justice underpins this practice, as mothers who find themselves in this situation are mostly facing complex intersections of social, economic, gendered, ableist and racist pressures and histories within their family experiences.

The process of removing a baby from its mother is also often at odds with the women-centred practice of midwives as noted by several researchers (Everitt, 2013; Marsh et al., 2019; Wood, 2008), their research on midwives' experiences found that being involved in the removal of a baby was a negative challenge to the 'midwife-woman' relationship. Research also found that midwives were aware of their role in causing bereavement by participating in the removal of a child (Wood, 2008). The loss of a baby who is removed at birth mirrors the loss of a stillborn baby, but the grief is not always recognised, and according to the midwives in Wood's (2008) study, they were not supported in the same way, observing that such women are discharged without the same follow-up for their loss. Further, according to Everitt (2013) midwives indicated that being involved in the actual removal of babies negatively challenged the midwife–woman relationship. This was connected to knowing that being a midwife is to be 'with woman' and was an intrinsic ethos for the midwife–woman relationship (Everitt, 2013).

Feminist Medical Doctors

Feminist medical doctors are also involved in feminist practice concerned with women's welfare in reproductive medicine. On a website 'Feminism in India' (FII), Dr Suchitra Dalvie, has made a post as part of a campaign entitled 'Health Over Stigma' about women's experiences of gynaecology both in training as specialist doctors but with a focus on patients' experiences. Dr Dalvie stated at the outset:

> As a practicing feminist gynaecologist, I wanted to offer a glimpse of what this world looks like from the other side of the consulting table/examination bed.
>
> *(FII, 2019)*

In her blog, she described her experience as a student where she observed high levels of misogynistic practices by senior male gynaecologists, including abusing women's bodies while under anaesthetic, conducting abortions on young women without an anaesthetic as a form of punishment, high levels of sexist abuse of female students and a complete lack of reference to gender equality, feminism and misogyny in her education. As a practitioner she went on the be a feminist activist, promoting and ensuring feminist informed practices, with a focus on abortion access. Reflecting the global problem of medicine's dominance by men and patriarchal frameworks, the following is a statement from a Canadian neuro-science student, Sara El Jaouhari (2021) reflecting her view of the intersectional challenges in studying medicine:

> It must be emphasized, however, that any discussion of gender requires a discussion of race, power, privilege, and identity, all of which are intricately linked. Moreover, we must recognize the role that medicine has played as an institution in perpetuating systemic racism and sexism. As providers, we understand that gender is a social determinant of health; the link between gender bias and poor health outcomes in patients is well established. We also know that a diverse workforce, including racialized women, enhances patient care and improves health outcomes. By advocating for gender equity as a health matter, we can serve as powerful agents of change. We can start by looking critically at the policies that contribute to gender inequity within our own profession.

There is evidence that research is seeking to transform medical practices that lead to sexism and gendered oppression in treatment through transforming the education of doctors (Sharma, 2019). As an educator and practitioner, Malika Sharma made the following observations:

> Trainees learn mostly about male diagnosticians and scientists, in academic institutions where men take up most leadership positions. This historical gendering of medicine prioritises particular types of knowledge (and ways of producing that knowledge), and creates barriers for critical, and specifically feminist, research and practice. Patriarchy has ripple effects, such as harassment, the gender wage gap, and gender segregation in specialties and medical leadership.
>
> *(2019, p. 570)*

Sharma's observations about medical education in Canada are widely applicable across the world. She went on to note that the absence of feminist theory in teaching medicine suggested 'that academic institutions continue to create a culture of medicine and medical education that is rooted in patriarchy, with the perspectives of women, and especially women of colour, pushed to the margins' (Sharma, 2019, p. 576). The way medicine is taught clearly informs practice, but it is evident that medical practice can be feminist, there is simply a very long way to go to transform all medical practice and consequently improve the experiences of women and transgender men in medical care and institutions.

Conclusion

There is a myriad of ways and means of abuse, violence and control over women and transgender men through social, legal, and medical constructions and processes of reproduction, motherhood, maternity, and childbirth. In these universal spheres of social welfare, there are powerful convergences of sexism, racism, elitism and judgement about class and culture. It is one of the most important sites for feminist practice and confronts the depths of persistent and diverse forms of patriarchal control and knowledge. Although the areas of motherhood and other's childbirth experiences and context covered in this chapter are wide ranging, they are not complete as a representation of the ways that feminist practice has or should intervene to ensure social justice in this field. From a global perspective, there are many other experiences that women endure in their positions of maternity. The aim here was to provide some insight into how feminist practice has intervened, resisted, analysed or established greater agency for those in childbirth and their experiences as mothers or transgender men who choose to have children. Maternal morbidity and health are key global social welfare measures for communities and nations and reflect underlying policy principles for gender equality. In the following chapter, the broader terrain of reproductive welfare and rights is the focus.

References

AIHW (Australian Institute of Health and Welfare) (2017) *Maternal Deaths in Australia 2012–2014*. Canberra: Australian Government. https://www.aihw.gov.au/reports/mothers-babies/maternal-deaths-in-australia-2012-2014/contents/risk-factors-for-maternal-death.

AIHW (Australian Institute of Health and Welfare) (2019) *The Health of Australia's Prisoners 2018*. Canberra: AIHW. https://www.aihw.gov.au/reports/prisoners/health-australia-prisoners-2018/contents/summary.

Alptraum, L. (2017) bell hooks on the state of feminism and how to move forward under Trump: BUST interview. *Bust* (Online magazine). https://bust.com/feminism/19119-the-road-ahead-bell-hooks.html.

Anolack, H. (2015) Our bodies, our choice: Australian law and foetal personhood. *Women and Birth*, 28, 60–64.

Atuahene, M.D., Arde-Acquah, S., Atuahene, N.F., et al. (2017) Inclusion of men in maternal and safe motherhood services in inner-city communities in Ghana: Evidence from a descriptive cross-sectional survey. *BMC Pregnancy Childbirth*, 17, 419 (Online). https://bmcpregnancychildbirth.biomedcentral.com/articles/10.1186/s12884-017-1590-3#citeas.

BBC News (2018) Single mothers hit hard by homelessness. October 10, 2018. https://www.bbc.com/news/uk-45800186.

Bielefeld, S. (2012) Compulsory income management and indigenous Australians: Delivering social justice or furthering colonial domination. *UNSW Law Journal*, 35 (2), 522–562.

Boerma, T., Ronsmans, C., Melesse, D.Y., et al. (2019) Global epidemiology of use of and disparities in caesarean sections. *The Lancet*, 398 (10155), 1341–1348.

Briggs, L. (2017) *How All Politics became Reproductive Politics: From Welfare Reform to Foreclosure to Trump.* Berkeley: University of California Press.

Bringing Them Home Report (1997) *Report of the National Inquiry into the Separation of Aboriginal and Torres Strait Islander Children from Their Families April 1997.* Human Rights Commission: Australian Government https://www.humanrights.gov.au/publications/bringing-them-home-report-1997.

Brooks, K. (2018) America is blaming pregnant women for their own deaths. *The New York Times*, November 16, 2018. https://www.nytimes.com/2018/11/16/opinion/sunday/maternal-mortality-rates.html.

Cacciatore, J. and Wieber Lens, J. (2019) The ultimate in women's labor: Stillbirth and grieving. In J. Ussher, J. Chrisler and J. Perz (eds) *Routledge International Handbook of Women's Sexual and Reproductive Health.* Oxon; New York: Routledge, 308–318.

Campoamor, L. (2016) "Who are you calling exploitative?" Defensive motherhood, child labor, and urban poverty in Lima, Peru. *The Journal of Latin American and Caribbean Anthropology*, 21 (1), 151–172.

Center for Disease Control and Prevention (2018) Pregnancy Mortality Surveillance System (Updated August 2018) https://www.cdc.gov/reproductivehealth/maternalinfanthealth/pregnancy-mortality-surveillance-system.htm

Chaturvedi, S., De Costa, A. and Raven, J. (2015). Does the Janani Suraksha Yojana cash transfer programme to promote facility births in India ensure skilled birth attendance? A qualitative study of intrapartum care in Madhya Pradesh. *Global Health Action*, 8 (1), 27427.

Clarke, A. (2010) The second-hand brand: liquid assets and borrowed goods. In D. Wengrow and A. Bevan (eds) *Cultures of Commodity Branding.* Walnut Creek, CA: Left Coast Press, 235–254.

Clarke, A. (2014) Designing mothers and the market: Social class and maternal culture. In S. O'Donohoe, M. Hogg, P. Maclaren, L. Martens and L. Stevens (eds) *Mothers, Markets and Consumption, The Making of Mother in Contemporary Western Cultures.* London; New York: Routledge, 43–55.

Coast, C., Jones, E., Lattof, S.R. and Portela, A. (2016). Effectiveness of interventions to provide culturally appropriate maternity care in increasing uptake of skilled maternity care: A systematic review. *Health Policy and Planning*, 31 (10), 1479–1491.

Curtis, C.M. and Denby, R.W. (2004) Impact of the Adoption and Safe Families Act (1997) on families of color: Workers share their thoughts. *Families in Society*, 85 (1), 71–79.

Dixon, L.Z. (2015) Obstetrics in a time of violence: Mexican midwives critique of routine hospital practices. *Medical Anthropology Quarterly*, 29 (4), 437–454.

D'Gregorio, R.P. (2010) Obstetric violence: A new legal term introduced in Venezuela. *International Journal of Gynecology and Obstetrics*, 111, 201–202. http://www.redehumanizasus.net/sites/default/files/figo_-_violencia_obstetrica_-_legislacao_na_venezuela.pdf.

Douglas, V. (2006). Childbirth among the Canadian Inuit: A review of the clinical and cultural literature. *International Journal of Circumpolar Health*, 65 (2), 117–132.

Dunkerley, S. (2017) Mothers matter: A feminist perspective on child welfare-involved women. *Journal of Family Social Work*, 20 (3), 251–265.

El Jaouhari, S. (2021) The ongoing need for feminism in medicine. *Canadian Medical Education Journal*, 12 (2), e118–e119.

Elliot, S. and Bowen, S. (2018) Defending motherhood: Morality, responsibility, and double binds in feeding children. *Journal of Marriage and Family*, 80 (2), 499–520.

Escude, M. and Law, V. (2013) My mom is badder than yours: Women prisoners demand better conditions for motherhood behind bars. *Wagadu*, 11, 9–19.

Everitt L. (2013) The experiences of midwives working with removal of newborns for child protection concerns in NSW, Australia: Being in the headspace and heartspace. Unpublished MSc Thesis, University of Technology, Sydney.

Evershed, N. and Allam, L. (2018) Indigenous children's removal on the rise 21 years after bringing them home. *The Guardian*, Australian Edition, May 2018. https://www.theguardian.com/australia-news/2018/may/25/australia-fails-to-curb-childrens-removal-from-indigenous-families-figures-show.

Fejo-King, C. (2011) The national apology to the stolen generations: The ripple effect. *Australian Social Work*, 64 (1), 130–143.

FII (Feminism in India) (2019) Being a feminist gynaecologist in the patriarchal world of medicine. *#MyGynaecStory*. https://feminisminindia.com/2019/11/19/feminist-gynaecologist-patriarchal-medicine/.

Fonseca, C. (2002) The politics of adoption: Child rights in the Brazilian setting. *Law & Policy*, 24 (3), 199–227.

Gil, S. (2017) *Obstetric Violence and Human Rights in Brazil: What happened, Mrs Adelir de Goés?* London School of Economics, LSE Human Rights: A student led blog from the Centre for the Study of Human Rights. http://blogs.lse.ac.uk/humanrights/2017/02/06/obstetric-violence-and-human-rights-in-brazil-what-happened-mrs-adelir-de-goes/.

Goodwin, S. and Huppatz, K. (2010) *The Good Mother: Contemporary Motherhoods in Australia*. Sydney: Sydney University Press.

Gopichandran, V., Subramaniam, S. and Kalsingh, M.J. (2018) Psycho-social impact of stillbirths on women and their families in Tamil Nadu, India – A qualitative study. *BMC Pregnancy and Childbirth*, 18 (109), 1–13.

Governor Phil Murphy (2021) New Jersey first lady Tammy Murphy unveils ground-breaking plan to eliminate racial disparities in New Jersey's maternal and infant mortality. *State of New Jersey Governor Phil Murphy*, January 25. https://www.nj.gov/governor/news/news/562021/20210125a.shtml.

Gunnersson Payne, J. and Erbenius, T. (2018) Conceptions of transgender parenthood in fertility care and family planning in Sweden: From reproductive rights to concrete practices. *Anthropology and Medicine*, 25 (3), 329–343.

Hattenstone, S. (2019) Father and son. *The Guardian Weekly*, 200 (20) (April 26, 2019), 10–14.

Hosseine, S. (2019) The buzz about Meghan Markle's birth plan has highlighted the stigma around home births. *The Washington Post*, May 3. https://www.washingtonpost.com/lifestyle/2019/05/03/buzz-about-meghan-markles-birth-plan-has-highlighted-stigma-around-home-births/.

IJRC (International Justice Resource Centre) (2017) IACTHR holds Bolivia responsible for forced sterilization in landmark judgment (Posted January 3, 2017). https://ijrcenter.org/2017/01/03/iacthr-holds-bolivia-responsible-for-forced-sterilization-in-landmark-judgment/.

Jackson, M.K., Schmied, V. and Dahlen, H.G. (2020) Birthing outside the system: The motivation behind the choice to freebirth or have a homebirth with risk factors in Australia. *BMC Pregnancy Childbirth*, 20, 254.

Khan, M.E., Hazra, A. and Bhatnagar, I. (2010) Impact of Janani Suraksha Yojana on selected family health behaviours in rural Uttar Pradesh. *The Journal of Family Welfare*, 56 (Special Issue), 9–22.

Kuleshova, A. (2015) Dilemmas of modern motherhood (based on research in Russia). *Economics and Sociology*, 8 (4), 110–121.

Leap, N. (2009) Woman-centred or women-centred care: Does it matter? *British Journal of Midwifery*, 19 (1), 12–16.

Manne, A. (2018) Mothers and the quest for social justice, from the 'Universal Bread-winner' to the 'Universal Caregiver' regime. In C. Nelson and R. Roberson (eds) *Dangerous Ideas about Mothers*. Crawley: University of WA Publishing, 17–33.

Margaria, A. (2020) Trans men giving birth and reflections on fatherhood: What to expect? *International Journal of Law, Policy and the Family*, 34 (3), 225–246.

Marsh, W., Robinson, A., Gallagher, A. and Shawe, J. (2014). Removing babies from mothers at birth: Midwives' experiences. *British Journal of Midwifery*, 22 (9), 620–624.

MMM (Make Mothers Matter) (2017) Statement on international day on the elimina-tion of violence against women: Time to stop obstetric violence (Posted November 25, 2017). https://makemothersmatter.org/statement-on-international-day-on-the-elimination-of-violence-against-women-time-to-stop-obstetric-violence/.

Nelson, C. and Robertson, R. (2018) What's behind the rise of Mummy Bullies? In C. Nelson and R. Roberson (eds) *Dangerous Ideas about Mothers*. Crawley: University of WA Publishing, 1–13.

OECD (2019) Caesarean sections (indicator). doi:10.1787/adc3c39f-en (Published 2017). (Accessed April 15, 2019). https://data.oecd.org/healthcare/caesarean-sections.htm.

Ollove, M. (2018) A shocking number of U.S. women still die of childbirth. Califor-nia is doing something about that. *The Washington Post*, November 4, 2018. https://www.washingtonpost.com/national/health-science/a-shocking-number-of-us-women-still-die-from-childbirth-california-is-doing-something-about-that/2018/11/02/11042036-d7af-11e8-a10f-b51546b10756_story.html?noredirect=on&utm_term=.4924025a.

Owen, L. and Razak, A. (2019) Why Chinese mothers turned away from C-sections. BBC World Service, March 2. https://www.bbc.com/news/world-asia-china-46265808.

Payne, L. (2010) Toward the development of culturally safe birth models among northern First Nations: The Sioux Lookout Meno Ya Win Health Centre experience. Master of Public Health, Thesis. Simon Fraser University. http://summit.sfu.ca/item/11334.

Phillips, R. (2017) Women's poverty: Risks and experiences of poverty for Australian women. In K. Serr (ed.) *Thinking about Poverty* (4th ed.). Annandale: Federation Press, 137–147.

Rawlings, L. (1998) Traditional aboriginal birthing issues. *The Birth Gazette*, Summertown, 14 (1). https://www.proquest.com/docview/203154937?parentSessionId=4Ss8%2Ft FpLlT6oAZebxy%2BrUfWddvS%2FNOLYRwlhsQPNQs%3D&pq-origsite= primo&accountid=14757.

Riggs, D.W., Due, C. and Tape, N. (2018) Australian heterosexual men's expe-riences of pregnancy loss: The relationships between grief, psychological dis-tress, stigma, help-seeking, and support. *OMEGA-J Death Dying*. https://doi.org/10.1177/0030222818819339.

Sharma, M. (2019) Applying feminist theory to medical education. *The Lancet*, 393 (10171), 570–578.

Smith-Oka, V. (2013) Managing labor and delivery among impoverished populations in Mexico: Cervical examinations as bureaucratic practice. *American Anthropologist*, 115 (4), 595–607.

Summers, H. (2020) Women feel they have no option but to give birth alone: The rise of freebirthing. *The Guardian*, Saturday, December 5. https://www.theguardian.com/lifeandstyle/2020/dec/05/women-give-birth-alone-the-rise-of-freebirthing.

Syal, R. (2019) Benefit cap: Single mothers make up 85% of those affected, data shows. *The Guardian*, Australia Edition, Friday, January 4. https://www.theguardian.com/society/2019/jan/04/benefit-cap-single-mothers-make-up-85percent-of-those-affected-data-shows.

Tedmanson, D. and Fejo-King, C. (2016) Talking up and listening well, dismantling whiteness and building reflexivity. In S. Wendt and N. Moulding (eds) *Contemporary Feminisms in Social Work Practice* (1st ed.), 149–165. Routledge.

UNFPA (United Nations Population Fund) (2017) Worlds apart, reproductive rights in the age of inequality. *UNFPA State of the World's Population*. https://esaro.unfpa.org/en/publications/worlds-apart-reproductive-health-and-rights-age-inequality.

UN Women (2017) UN Women and the World Bank unveil new data analysis on women and poverty. UN Women Website. http://www.unwomen.org/en/news/stories/2017/11/news-un-women-and-the-world-bank-unveil-new-data-analysis-on-women-and-poverty.

Walker, J., Baldry, W. and Sullivan, E. (2019) Babies and toddlers are living with their mums in prison. We need to look after them better. *The Conversation*, May 17. https://theconversation.com/babies-and-toddlers-are-living-with-their-mums-in-prison-we-need-to-look-after-them-better-117170.

WHO (World Health Organization) (2018) *Maternal Mortality* (Last updated February 2018). https://www.who.int/news-room/fact-sheets/detail/maternal-mortality.

WHO (World Health Organization) (2013) Trends in caesarean delivery by country and wealth quintile: Cross-sectional surveys in southern Asia and sub-Saharan Africa. *Bulletin of the World Health Organization* (Last updated & published August 9). https://www.who.int/bulletin/volumes/91/12/13-117598/en/.

Wood, G. (2008) Taking the baby away removing babies at birth for safeguarding and child protection. *MIDIRS Midwife Digest*, 18 (3), 311–319.

5

REPRODUCTIVE JUSTICE, RIGHTS AND WELFARE, THE ROLE OF FEMINIST PRACTICE

Introduction

Although directly related to the terrain of motherhood and childbirth rights and experiences, as discussed in the last chapter, reproductive rights present a complex interplay between women's agency over their bodies and societal, religious, cultural and political impositions on the role of women as reproductive units. Mary Daly (1978) in *Gyn/Ecology: the metaethics of radical feminism*, details the violent misogynistic, biomedical past for women and midwives in most Western cultures. Beginning with 'wise women/healers' being executed as witches and the rise of men-midwives and its evolution into gynaecology from the 16th to the 19th century. Early in the 19th century, the practice of gynaecology, 'the science of women', was completely dominated by men, in keeping with an extreme male dominance of the female sex, where they brutally experimented by cutting up women's bodies to control and oppress women (Daly, 1978, pp. 225–226). For example:

> Clitoridectomy "invented" ten years later by the English gynecologist Isaac Baker Brown, was enthusiastically accepted as a "cure" for female masturbation by some American gynecologists [performed well into the 20th Century]. In 1852 Dr. Augustus Kinsley Gardner let out a battle cry against "disorderly women", including women's rightists, Bloomer-wearers [loose fit underwear that allowed freedom of movement, invented by women's rights activist, Amelia Jenks Bloomer], and midwives. In the 1860s Dr. Isaac Ray and his contemporaries proclaimed that women are susceptible to hysteria, insanity, and criminal impulses by reason of their sexual organs. The year 1872 marked the publication of Dr. Robert Battey's

DOI: 10.4324/9781315625188-5

invention of the "female castration", that is the removal of the ovaries to cure "insanity". For the next several decades ovariotomy became the gynecological craze; it was claimed to elevate the moral sense of the patients, making them tractable, orderly, industrious, and cleanly. "Disorderly" women were handed over to gynecologists by husbands and fathers for castration and other radical forms of treatment.

(Daly, 1978, pp. 227–228)

The history of the medicalisation of women's bodies underpins, it seems, many contemporary practices (as discussed in the previous chapter related to obstetric abuse) and restraints on women's bodily autonomy. Although the extreme nature of the historical practices described by Daly (1978) is no longer widespread, and many gynaecologists are now women, the struggle for women's self-determination over their reproductive capacity continues to be an issue for women's health and social welfare and must continue to be a focus for feminist practice.

The availability of new medical technologies for self-determining when, whether or how to have a child and even the capacity to select the gender of a child, have been at the centre of women's movement concerns and are firmly placed on feminist agendas across the world. This was recognised by the global women's movement in 1995 when, at the United Nations Fourth World Conference on Women in Beijing, the conference elevated reproductive health as a centrally important issue for women's human rights (Alzate, 2009). At the same time, the International Federation of Social Workers recognised reproductive health and rights as central to the philosophical foundation and practice of social work and as a core aspect of good social work practice, seeing such rights as intersecting with 'health, development, and human rights' (Alzate, 2009, p. 109). In this chapter feminist perspectives and practice related to key experiences of reproduction and how it relates to women's and others with reproductive capacity's rights and welfare will be discussed. Like in previous chapters, examples from around the world will be drawn upon to reflect the ubiquity of sexist views of women's reproductive capacity, but also the newer complexities of non-binary and transgender people and their engagement with reproduction. In examining feminist practices related to reproductive rights it is important to see reproduction as a form of agency that is owned and controlled by the bearer of that capacity, to recognise that as a right it can be chosen, restrained or denied by the bearer of reproductive capacity and therefore not be imposed upon or controlled as a form of oppression. Reproduction and the capacity to reproduce are deeply personal possessions or owned experiences. At the same time, they are often externalised as a highly political issues and sought to be controlled by institutional, political, religious, legal, social and traditional practices. This chapter will focus on social welfare in the form of rights, health, and safety in relation to the specific areas of menstruation, contraception, abortion, assisted reproduction and surrogacy.

Menstruation

The female capacity to reproduce has always been a touchpoint for girls' and women's oppression. There is ample evidence that throughout history and in the contemporary world it has been seen by leaders and decision-makers (who have been and *are* mostly men) and men in intimate partnerships with women as, on the one hand, an essential human role. On the other hand, it is seen as something that must be controlled or regulated. Medicalisation, violence, and ridicule have been instruments of oppression used against women's reproductive power in most cultural and social contexts. Although in some cultures, and within politically progressive communities, fertility and its attendant experiences are a celebration of emerging womanhood and fertility.

More commonly, discrimination, negativity and stigmatisation about menstruation are part of the shame of being a woman imposed on girls and women (Johnston-Robledo and Chrisler, 2020). Shame and insults are imposed by men, boys and some women brought up in repressive, mostly religious cultures. In those contexts, menstruation is seen as a corruption, as 'dirty' or as a curse. The visceral state of regular monthly bleeding has been constructed as an aberration in most societies, even though it is recognised as a normal biological process to facilitate fertility. In some cultural practices, women face exclusion and isolation during menstruation as well as cultural and religious rules where women are banned from temples, churches and public places and denied sexual encounters.

At the extreme end of such practices is a tradition in the Chhaupadi culture of Nepal, which requires women to isolate themselves, to live outside their home in an animal shed or a hut during their menstruation period (Ranabhat et al., 2015). They also face other restrictions such as the consumption 'of milk products; restricted access to public water sources; not being allowed to touch men, children, cattle, living plants, or fruit bearing trees' (Ranabhat et al., 2015, p. 786). This widespread practice was found to have profound physical and mental health implications for women in Nepal. Although acknowledging that there have been few studies on menstruation, Ranabhat et al. (2015) found that the practice of Chhaupadi might be a major cultural factor responsible for poor women's health status in Nepal. There were established links between the practice and low body weight of women and poor child health at twice the rate of the rest of the population as small children live in the huts with women during their period. Other health consequences included 'genital infections due to lack of menstrual hygiene, undernutrition due to some food barriers, and uterus and cervical problems due to heavy working, and recurrent infection of human papillomavirus as even though Chhaupadi does not directly cause any disease or illness, it facilitates an unsafe menstruation' (Ranabhat et al., 2015, p. 787). Studies also suggest that due to 'isolation, substance abuse, and stigmatization', it increases behavioural problems (Ranabhat et al., 2015, p. 787).

Part of the work of creating safe environments for young women in particular is to see menstruation as a normative experience relates to language. According to an online survey across 190 countries (*n*90,000) conducted by an online women's magazine, *Her*, there are 5,000 different ways for women and girls to express that they are menstruating (Her, 2017). As most terms are obscure euphemisms, there is still extensive discomfort in discussing, or even mentioning, menstruation. This is directly related to the stigma attached to the bodily process and as noted by Yomi Adegoke, an advocate for young people. She stated:

> All around the world girls, women, transgender, and intersex people suffer from the stigma of menstruation through bullying, cultural taboos, discrimination, and the inability to afford sanitary products – known as period poverty.
>
> *(Her, 2017)*

Plan International (2019), reported that in Uganda 28 per cent of girls miss school when they have their period and that in the Solomon Islands, 63 per cent of women can't afford sanitary pads. They also reported that 'period poverty' is evident in remote Indigenous communities because of the high price of menstrual hygiene products (Plan International, 2019). In the global North in particular, in the 2000s, there has been a gradual growth in 'menstruation liberation', where feminist activists have adopted menstruation activism. Organisations such as 'Bloody Good Period' have a mission to 'fight for menstrual equity and the rights for all people who bleed' (Good Bloody Period, 2021). They supply menstrual products for people who cannot afford them, provide education, 'normalise' mensuration, host an informative blog and hold rallies about access and ending period shame. The NGO supports other activities such as a Decolonising Menstruation workshops that aimed 'to create menstrual equity and end period shame, focused within the unique circumstances of Black, Indigenous and People of Colour … communities in England and Wales' (Good Bloody Period, 2021). Their activities reflect an intersectional approach, seeking to be inclusive of all groups of people who experience menstrual issues, including refugees and making links with women and girls in countries where there are high levels of stigma. Other types of feminist menstruation action included the organisation of a petition through social media to provide free menstrual products in schools in the UK.

More radical actions are also emerging, such as Kirin Ghandi who 'free-bled' when she ran the London Marathon in 2015 and posted a photograph on social media after the race that soon went viral. To create a political, period positive opportunity, she stated:

> It is so shocking for us as a society to see menstrual blood. That is why it trended on Twitter and Facebook for four days. It was so polarising," [and] 'The first criticism was that this is so gross, which was fine, because that was exactly the point: menstruation is still seen as something that's disgusting, even though it is the very thing that gives life to all of us'.
>
> *(Radnor, 2017)*

As a result of this type of activism and the broader embrace of the idea by fourth-wave feminists, there is now a commonly understood movement for 'period positivity' that challenges the deeply negative representations of menstruation. However, it should be recognised that second-wave feminists in the 1970s also deeply explored and challenged similar reactions and oppressions about menstruation through art and activism (Nelson, 2019) and although any generalised experience attributed to women (essentialising their sex) has been a criticism of the second wave, their projects were not dissimilar to current fourth wave activism and politics as the women's health movement made key demands to recognise specific health needs of women.

Feminist practice in this area has pointed to the importance of reproductive education for boys and girls. It is important to make connections between menstruation and reproduction, after all without it humans cannot reproduce naturally. It is also important for caregivers or parents to ensure that when a daughter begins menstruation it is not a shock or an embarrassment as this could be the beginning of a sense of inferiority intrinsically related to her gender, ensuring a secondary status compared to boys and men who do not go through the experience of what is seen as an affliction. In many cultures and societies, the physical and mental impact of menstruation (hormonal changes, mood changes and pain) have added to sexist shaming and jokes about women. Often a woman's period is used as an explanation for certain behaviours, if women stand up for themselves, are assertive, show emotion or are angry or upset they are insulted by being accused of menstruating – with expression like being 'on the rag' or suffering 'PMS' (premenstrual syndrome). This was elevated to a form of legitimate criticism of women in power when in 2008 on Fox News in the USA Bill O'Reilly asked a guest, Marc Rudolph, what the downside of having a woman in the Oval Office might be and he replied, 'You mean besides the PMS and the mood swings' (Grate, 2012). As noted by Rachel Grate (2012) if you Google PMS jokes, there are more than 4 million pages of results, demonstrating the extent to which women's menstruation has been vilified. In some cultures, oppressive views of menstruation are systematically applied, affecting social engagement and day-to-day freedoms. For example:

> Menstrual taboos have a major impact on women and girls in India, especially when they are young and are taught to 'discipline' their bodies and 'manage' menstruation according to certain norms. Taboos such as not entering the temple, sleeping on the floor, staying in separate rooms, eating in isolation, not touching holy things, not interacting with other members of the family, not touching anybody, and so on regulate twelve weeks of a woman's life every year.
>
> *(arora, 2017, p. 529)*

Along with the experience of living with menstruation is the inevitable end of the experience through menopause. Like menstruation, most women go through 'the change' silently and often, but not always, suffer due to dramatic hormonal changes in their bodies. The unspoken nature of menopause and its precursor, perimenopause, is a continuation of the societal negativity about menstruation but added to the invisibility of middle-aged women. As noted by Ilona Voicu (2018), biomedicalisation of menopause has constructed it as a disease that women should live in fear of, as the menopausal woman is seen as a 'useless body'. This idea is inherently sexist as it is often suggested that men retain their biological capacity to reproduce until they die, even though ageing does have a significant impact on male fertility and physical ability to be sexually active. Dr Jennifer Gunter, an outspoken feminist gynaecologist, observed when 'an idealized cis-gender male body is used as a so-called standard, it's easy to view the female body as flawed. This is a core tenet of the patriarchy' (Wiseman, 2019). This fear has become particularly the case in more recent decades as a result of the generalised resistance to anything that signifies ageing and as noted by Utz (2011, p. 143) 'major social institutions, including the media and pharmaceutical industry, have played a significant role in reshaping the cultural lens through which women experience issues of health, body, and aging'. Eun-Ok Im (2007), a nursing researcher, outlined how feminist activists had assisted women to move away from the regular medicalise responses to menopausal women's experiences of the range of effects of menopause, towards a self-managed model. She observed:

> …despite the widely suggested use of hormone therapy for vasomotor symptoms by healthcare providers, women themselves choose to manage their symptoms through self-care methods such as taking over-the-counter herbal products and vitamins, modifying their environment, and changing their behaviour rather than take hormones. Also, women themselves discuss menopause positively.
>
> *(Im, 2007, p. S15)*

Despite this movement, which has had some success in influencing health professionals and even legislation, the overwhelming response to menopause is medicalised. However, feminist medical professionals and researchers have begun to produce accessible books that seek to address women's experiences and fears and to normalise menopause. Experiences of perimenopause, something that is often an out-of-the-blue experience, commonly experienced as sudden, intense bleeding, was something I knew nothing about until another woman of a similar age described her experience; otherwise I think I would have thought I was about to die when struck with a flood of bleeding in transit from one country to another! Increasingly women are speaking out about such experiences, and it is often met with surprise that it is a shared experience (Hinsliff, 2021). Dr Jen Gunter's book *The Menopause Manifesto, Own Your Health with Facts and Feminism* is one such text that seeks to shift views about menopause, reframing it not a disease but as a planned change, like puberty. She calls for a planned approach that requires early education about what to expect rather than the current situation of most women left to cope with their symptoms and a wide range of conflicting advice. Her work, as a feminist gynaecologist seeks to empower and reassure women (Gunter, 2019).

Contraception and Rights to Abortion

The legal aspects of abortion are discussed in detail in Chapter 7 of this book. In this chapter, the right to determine one's own fertility is discussed, as well as key social welfare issues that arise when women and girls are denied support and assistance in determining their relationship to their own fertility. Contraception and abortion are interrelated by the risk of and the experience of an unintended pregnancy. According to Troutman et al. (2020), an unintended pregnancy is 'any unplanned, mistimed or unwanted pregnancy at the time of conception' and is a major public health problem as well at a fundamental reproductive right.

In a global study, it was estimated that there were 121 million unintended pregnancies annually in the world between 2015 and 2019, translating to a 'global rate of 64 unintended pregnancies' per 1,000 women between 15 and 49 years old (Bearak et al., 2020). Of those some 61 per cent ended in abortion, estimated as 73·3 million abortions annually (Bearak et al., 2020). The researchers found that in countries where access to abortion was restricted, rates of abortion 'had increased compared with the proportion for 1990–1994, and the unintended pregnancy rates were higher than in countries where abortion was broadly legal' (Bearak et al., 2020). This was evident in the level of reduction in abortions over the 30-year period, which meant a reduction of 63 per cent in Europe and North America, less so in Australia and New Zealand at 19 per cent and even less in West Asia and North Africa (by 14 per cent) (Bearak et al., 2020). Bearak et al. (2020) noted that increased availability of contraception and access to family planning services cannot guarantee a reduced number of unintended pregnancies but recognised that family planning programmes had led to an increase in contraceptive use. Factors, such as the availability of long-acting reversible contraception (LARC), which is a group of contraception methods that provide very effective, long acting and reversible contraception, access to family planning services and general contraceptive education, have contributed to women's greater reproductive autonomy and a reduction in unplanned pregnancies.

Feminist activism and practice have been at the heart of providing access to contraceptives since the 1970s, when second-wave feminists took direct action to secure women's reproductive rights. An example of such action was when a group called Irish Women United (IWU) set up the Contraception Action Program (CAP), which opened a shop with the purpose of providing over-the-counter contraceptives to Irish women and challenging the prohibitive Irish law on contraceptives (Kelly, 2019). Although the shop was instantly successful and was not raided by police for transgressing contraceptive law, it closed within two years due to ideological differences (Kelly, 2019). However other important grassroots service organisations grew and developed from the group, 'including the first Rape Crisis Centre in 1977', and 'the Women's Right to Choose Group and the crisis pregnancy and abortion referral organisation, Open Line Counselling, were founded in 1979' (Kelly, 2019, p. 270). Laura Kelly's research with grassroots activist women from CAP noted the wider context for women in Ireland in the 1970s:

> Women living in 1970s Ireland suffered from a range of inequalities that had been in existence since the early-twentieth century, including lack of equal pay for equal work and the marriage bar whereby women who had a jobs in the public service had to give up their job upon marriage. Additionally, women could not sit on a jury until 1972 and could not own a home outright until 1976. Moreover, contraception had been illegal since 1935 under the Criminal Law Amendment Act, while the Censorship of Publications Act had banned the sale of literature relating to birth control since 1929. Contraception therefore became a 'unifying question...'
>
> *(2019, p. 274)*

The power of the Catholic Church in Ireland was a key target for feminist activists in their struggle for reproductive rights in Ireland. Many medical practitioners were highly influenced by Catholicism and feminists, in the Irish Women's Liberation Movement, confronted that power in various ways. This included 'walkouts from Catholic masses and protests at government buildings', and instigated the 'Contraceptive Train' stunt, in May 1971 (Kelly, 2019). Highlighting the hypocrisy of the Irish law, a group of women travelled to Belfast (where contraception was legal under U.K. law), purchased contraceptives and returned to Dublin, went through customs and were able to retain their purchases (Kelly, 2019, p. 274). In elaborating about the wider women's movement in the 1970s, Kelly pointed to worldwide concerns women had about the health impact of the most accessible contraceptive (given to lower-income women for free in Ireland) at that time, 'the pill' – expressing concerns about the experimental nature of a drug that was not 100 per cent effective, seen as widely over prescribed generally, and that 'women's reproductive healthcare had become over-medicalised' with insufficient information on side effects on women's health (2019, p. 281). It was not until the 1990s that condoms became legal in Ireland and other contraceptives became legal in 1993, this was decades later than in the UK, for example. The eventual successful access to contraception demonstrates the importance of feminist practice in the struggle for reproductive rights.

The World Health Organisation (WHO) has outlined many reasons for the effectiveness of globally available contraception, this includes the prevention of maternal morbidity as it: allows spacing of pregnancies; delaying pregnancies in young girls at increased risk of health problems and risk of poverty from early childbearing; and preventing pregnancies among older women facing increased health and poverty risks (WHO, 2019). Contraception gives women reproductive control within families, and reduces rates of unintended pregnancies and the need for unsafe abortions. It has a low cost, on average, approximately US$1.55 per user annually in 'developing countries' (WHO, 2019). The use of condoms is also effective at preventing the transmission of AIDS and other sexually transmitted diseases. It is clearly a social justice issue and central to many peoples' welfare where there is a lack of access to or information about contraception.

Despite the fundamental feminist argument that it should be a woman's right to choose to have an abortion, much of the ongoing legislative and policy debate focuses on nuances of laws protecting women from unsafe abortions and conditions on the viability of a foetus determining when it is acceptable to have an abortion. Framing the need for access to abortion as a broad social welfare issue, the WHO focused on the impact of laws, policies, health standards and guidelines:

> The association between restrictive abortion laws and unsafe abortion has been well documented. According to an analysis by UN DESA, the average rate of unsafe abortion is estimated to be more than four times higher in countries with more restrictive abortion laws than in countries with less restrictive laws. Restrictive abortion laws are also associated with higher levels of maternal mortality. The average maternal mortality ratio is three times higher in countries with more restrictive abortion laws (223 maternal deaths per 100 000 live births) compared to countries with less restrictive laws (77 maternal deaths per 100 000 live births). Restrictive legal grounds for abortion are only one of many policy barriers that affect women and girls' access to safe abortion. Other barriers include policies that limit provision of abortion care to obstetricians and gynaecologists working at high-level care facilities; conscientious objection by health-care providers; requirements for third-party authorization(s); unnecessary medical tests; mandatory counselling; and mandatory waiting periods.
>
> (Johnson et al., 2017)

According to a 2014 United Nations report on the world's abortion laws, there are direct relationships between highly restrictive abortion laws, high maternal mortality and high numbers of teenage pregnancies, as generally where abortion is restricted so too is access to family planning support and contraception. This is a core welfare issue that affects women directly and reflects how religious morality conflicts with feminist struggles for women's autonomy and rights to determine their own fertility.

What underlies this data about abortion, and the various legislative approaches, is that if abortion in an appropriate medical setting is not available to women or girls who choose and need to terminate an unplanned pregnancy, then they will take risks and proceed anyway. The WHO report goes on to point out that abortion laws and policies that restrict access to abortion 'create risks to women and girls' health' because they are deterred from getting appropriate support and provision of care within a formal health system (Johnson et al., 2017). History has shown that if women cannot get a safe abortion, for a range of reasons (such as poverty, too many children already, a need to continue working, being a victim of rape, not having a partner to assist in parenting, being too young to choose motherhood and so on) they will seek help outside the medically safe options, hence the 'unsafe abortion' practice. The other effect of abortion laws is to create administrative barriers or 'sociogeographic' barriers to access, which cause delays and places women at higher medical risks (Johnson, 2017). The WHO Report also noted that

> restrictions on access to safe abortion create inequalities both within and between countries, making access to safe abortion a privilege of the rich and leaving poor women little choice but to resort to illegal and usually unsafe practices and providers.
>
> *(Johnson et al., 2017)*

The corollary of these laws is that medical services that would provide terminations are hindered and restricted in what they can offer. Many abortion laws and policies are designed to appease people in communities and society more generally who are opposed to abortion on religious grounds and choose to place the life of a foetus above the rights of a woman. They are a powerful and often aggressive group and a generally aligned with fundamentalist Christians and political conservatives who are vocally anti-feminist. As O'Donnell observed of the USA,

> since legalization, there have been murders and arson committed against abortion providers. Antiabortion advocates have championed laws enacted at the state level that creatively restrict access to the procedure for many, subverting constitutional rights under the guise of protecting women.
>
> *(2017, p. 79)*

In Australia, where different states have differing legal approaches to abortion, although it is generally unrestricted despite the legislations in place, laws were introduced to require 'pro-life' activists to be excluded from no-protest zones around abortion clinics to prevent women from being harassed and intimidated, to protect their rights of access to abortion (ABC, 2019). This measure is the result of feminist activism that has held true to the principle of pro-choice, a woman's right to choose. This struggle was a core objective of the second wave and in her historical account of that struggle in the USA, O'Donnell described how the Abortion Counselling Service of the Chicago Women's Liberation Union, 'known colloquially as "Jane" after the pseudonym its members adopted', operated as an underground service for women seeking abortions (2017, p. 78). 'Jane' developed their own skills to perform safe abortions, providing a service to women of colour and poor women who would otherwise not be able to gain access to abortions. This early grassroots action formed the basis of an extensive network of women's health centres in countries in the global North, establishing counselling services to ensure women had accurate information.

Highlighting the contemporary power of the use of social media as feminist practice, responding to the assault on women's right to abortion in the USA in 2018, has been the establishment of an online campaign #YouKnowMe, which commenced after a talk show host Busy Phillipps spoke about her abortion experience, hence precipitating a way for other woman to tell of their experience and how having an abortion freed them from both short and long term limitations on their life choices (Safronova, 2019). As pointed out by Prendergast (2018) this was a contemporary version of action women, including Billy Jean King, Nora Ephron, Judy Collins and 50 other celebrities, took in 1972 when they placed an advertisement in *Ms*. Magazine entitled 'We all Had Abortions'. This type of feminist action steps outside the confrontational debates with 'pro-life' activists and religious institutions aiming to control what women do by utilising women's lived experiences, to build solidarity with other women who made the same autonomous choices.

As with most countries in the African continent, abortion in Kenya is only allowed when a mother's life and health is at risk or 'when a trained medical professional believes the situation to be an emergency' (Center for Reproductive Rights, 2019). The cultural context in Kenya creates a high level of stigmatisation and imposes shame on women who have an abortion, therefore women are forced into unsafe, underground abortions from untrained health providers. This results in 465,000 illegal abortions annually and a quarter of those end up with severe health complications and hospitalisation (Center for Reproductive Rights, 2019). Thousands of women and girls are injured for life – or do not survive (Center for Reproductive Rights, 2019). The following case study reflects the severe impact of a system that does not support reproductive rights:

> In the Kenyan context, *Wanjiku* is symbolic of an ordinary person—any woman, every woman—and in a country where more than 30 percent of girls under 18 experience sexual violence and more than 40 percent of pregnancies are unintentional, Wanjiku's story represents the stories of hundreds of thousands just like her.
>
> When she was just 14, Wanjiku was coerced into a sexual relationship with an older man in her village and later discovered that she was pregnant. Abortion is stigmatized in Kenya due to conservative religious beliefs, and Wanjiku found herself in a desperate situation with no way out. Like many other women and girls who find themselves in this position, Wanjiku sought abortion care from an unqualified provider. She became ill almost immediately after the procedure and required immediate medical attention. Instead, she had to visit multiple hospitals that could not provide the necessary services. When she finally did find a qualified facility, she was neglected, abused, and forced to sleep on a mattress on the dirty hospital floor during her stay.

In 2015, the Center for Reproductive Rights filed a petition to hold the government accountable for this gross injustice. The petition challenges the lack of guidelines on abortion that can guide health care providers in cases such as Wanjiku's. The petition further challenges the government's directive banning health providers from participating in any abortion training thus limiting their ability to respond in cases where abortion is necessary or where post abortion care is required. By withdrawing the Standards and Guidelines for reducing morbidity and mortality from unsafe abortions in Kenya, prohibiting trainings on safe abortion care, and banning medabon, a safe and effective method of medication abortion, the Kenyan government stole Wanjiku's life. The Center has been fighting for Wanjiku and her mother for almost four years now. For Three years after the petition was filed, and after suffering from a slew of severe health complications for over four years as a result of the botched procedure, Wanjiku passed away. The Center has been fighting for Wanjiku and her mother for almost four years now, and for those four years, Wanjiku suffered from a slew of severe health complications that could have been prevented if she had received timely care after the botched procedure. Ultimately, this delay in care led to her premature death …

(Centre for Reproductive Rights, 2019)

The narrative of Wanjiku's experience is not unique, as many women across the world have similar experiences and have had so for decades, which is why feminist struggles for the right to a medically safe, legal abortion have been central to the cause in many national contexts. An innovative program run by the Middle African Network for Women's Reproductive Health (GCG) in Gabon, which was based on a programme developed by feminists in the Caribbean, to train regional midwives and other medical practitioners to perform basic abortion procedures, was developed for the local context (Ndembi Ndembi et al., 2019). In Gabon, contraception was illegal from 1969 to 2000 and abortions had become a common contraceptive alternative despite it being illegal. The researcher/activists noted that in Gabon, one in eighty-five women of reproductive age was at high risk of dying from pregnancy-related complications, including post-abortion illness. The researcher/activists focused on one region when they recruited midwives and other medical practitioners to begin the program. They reported:

Participants expounded on the main health risks of pregnancy, namely infection, haemorrhage, hypertension, and severe anaemia, which are often compounded by conditions such as HIV, malaria, tuberculosis, and diabetes. They enumerated the lacunas in material conditions, including light, water, electricity, sterile gloves, stethoscopes, telephones, transportation, incubators, oxygen, a blood bank, and contraceptives. In addition, they bemoaned the obstacles faced by women in accessing services (stemming from a lack of money and transportation), together with those that they, as service providers, faced in administering emergency care (due to inadequate equipment and skills). They expressed relief at the presence of an international team led by someone from their own community (midwife Mekuí was born in Bitam and speaks Fang) for the purpose of improving service delivery. We knew that although we could not resolve the infrastructural needs, we could improve the emergency care that was currently being offered.

(Ndembi Ndembi et al., 2019, p. 148)

Since the training began in 2009, which was carried out in neighbouring Tunis where abortion was legal, the GCG successfully trained 500 midwives to carry out the simple procedures that were effectively used to address health problems that arose from attempted abortions (as well as miscarriages and other pregnancy problems) (Ndembi Ndembi et al., 2019). This example of feminist praxis demonstrates how broad social welfare is an integral aspect of supporting women's health. The lack of resources beyond large hospitals is a common social policy problem across the world; in this case, the prevention of post-partum complications after abortions could be addressed by the performance of immediate interventions by locally trained midwives (Ndembi Ndembi et al., 2019). The GCG activist/researchers made an important point about not being able to wait for legislative change to make abortion legal, as the health needs resulting from self-administered abortions were dire and required a radically different welfare approach, one that focussed on geographical need and a reliance on forming alliances with local health workers, in which they were able to show impressive, direct improvements for women's reproductive health (Ndembi Ndembi et al., 2019). This program demonstrates direct feminist praxis by health professionals, strategically designed to address areas of highest need, creating a social justice context that improved the welfare and health outcomes for women and their families. It also demonstrates feminist research practice that ensures that the model can be understood and adapted further in different contexts of high need.

Given that most forcibly displaced people in the world are women and children (Bendavid et al., 2021) reproductive rights, and access to abortion are severely affected during conflict and natural disaster. Although there is little specific research on what happens to women's reproductive needs during conflict, it is evident that 'women and children are vulnerable to sexual violence, early marriage, harassment, isolation, and exploitation' (Bendavid et al., 2021, p. 529). According to an extensive review of prior research, 21 per cent of women displaced by conflict 'experienced sexual violence, which is possibly an underestimate because of social stigma, poor law enforcement systems, and inadequate services' (Bendavid et al., 2021, p. 529).

Feminist medical practitioners and activists, therefore, play a crucial role in supporting women's reproductive rights during conflict. For example, during the 2022 Russian invasion of Ukraine, millions of civilians were forced to flee across neighbouring borders, including into Poland where the abortion laws deny most women access to abortion and have criminalised women for seeking and getting abortions. Feminist gynaecologist, Myroslava Marchenko had her practice in Kyiv, Ukraine, until she too was forced to flee to Poland and took on a role of providing critical reproductive advice (mostly to go somewhere else, such as Germany where abortion is legal) for women refugees from Ukraine who had already planned an abortion, required an abortion due to the impact of the war or were victims of rape (Liminowicz, 2022). Poland is ranked as the worst country in Europe for access to contraception and '[m]any doctors refuse to prescribe emergency contraception or even IUDs (intrauterine devices) on ethical grounds, arguing that they are akin to an abortion' (Liminowicz, 2022). Women crossing into Poland were met by local feminist activists offering support but also by anti-abortion activists, 'handing out leaflets at refugee reception points depicting dismembered foetuses and citing abortion as the biggest threat to peace. The leaflets also advised pregnant women to denounce to the police anyone offering them an abortion' (Liminowicz, 2022). This was balanced by the Polish feminist organisations assisting women with their reproductive needs. This situation demonstrates the highly political nature of women's reproductive rights and how easily they can disappear in times of conflict and upheaval.

Assisted Reproductive Technologies

For second-wave feminists, the advent of assisted reproductive technologies (ART) brought new fields of feminist theorising and political engagement. The varied theories included an early excitement about the potential for women's autonomy and a capacity to procreate without men, a kind of utopia that gave women complete control of their fertility and reproduction. Alison Caddick (1995) explained Shulamith Firestone's (1972) radical view as:

> …the mind-body "normative dualism" is asserted in the proposal that test-tube conception and gestation-tank technology will free women from a system of sex-class distinctions rooted in the biological body? Rather than this pointing to a future free of the oppression of women, women as such will disappear altogether. Indeed, Firestone wishes "not just to eliminate male privilege but the sex distinction itself…"
>
> *(1995, p. 144)*

This revolutionary view was tempered by other critical feminists who drew their analysis from an inherent distrust of the patriarchal medical establishment. For example, Gena Corea (1985) in her book *The Mother Machine: From Artificial Insemination to Artificial Wombs*, explored historical and new reproductive technologies with a focus on the sexual politics of practices, including insemination, embryo transfer, surrogate parenting, sex selection, in vitro fertilisation (IVF), as well as cloning. Her overall analysis proposed that reproductive technologies were medical mechanisms, for the social, medical and legal control of women's bodies (Corea, 1985). Many of the issues raised by Corea (1985) are still important concerns in the contemporary context and are often used to inform the law related to reproductive technologies. She asked question about the types of relationships and economic security that would emerge for children, with the capacity for single women and gay couples to have babies, the exploitation of women for their eggs and use in surrogacy in their attempts to survive economically, the huge costs and consequences of unequal access, and ethical issues arising from genetic screening and its potential eugenic implications (Corea, 1985).

As the technologies developed beyond the experimental (having emerged primarily from veterinary science) in the 1980s, a range of regulations were introduced, driven by social welfare concerns for children born from ARTs. This related to aspects such as poor practices in artificial insemination where secrecy about the genetic father was highly protected by medical practitioners mixing donors' sperm and failing to keep records. Having learned from adoption experiences of children and their genealogical bewilderment from not having any knowledge of their birth parents, laws were introduced to ensure children could gain knowledge about their genetic heritage. Other regulations related to the number of embryos that could be implanted as research into the relationship between IVF babies and pre-term birth, particularly for multiple child pregnancies, were linked to serious health issues for children. Medical research has also shown higher risks for the IVF mother, as demonstrated in a nation-wide population study on the USA that found that although the IVF pregnancies were only 17 per cent of the births (170,000 in 2014), and that the mothers were 'older, wealthier, Caucasian, non-smokers', many medical conditions were evident (Sabban et al., 2017). This included, among other medical conditions, high percentages of pre-eclampsia, gestational diabetes, antepartum haemorrhage, pre-term premature rupture of membranes, caesarean section, increased risk of post-partum haemorrhage and hysterectomy as well as needs for transfusion, prolonged hospitalisation and pre-term birth (Sabban et al., 2017, p. 108). The high risks of early practices prompted concerns about IVF as an experimental medicine and added to the advent of surrogacy as part of the ARTs offerings, the marketisation of children and the exploitation of women as surrogate mothers. I experienced these debates in the mid-1980s, first-hand, as part of the Western Australian Government's Reproductive Technology Council, which was set up to report to the government on how a regulatory framework should be established for reproductive technologies. What was very striking at the time, the mid-1980s, was the very low success rate of IVF procedures, making it a repeated and expensive process, and how often the Council heard claims from women and their partners to the *right* to have children. Ethical considerations were very much overshadowed by the advocacy for those seeking to address infertility. The concerns of radical feminists mentioned above, are in stark contrast to liberal feminists of the second wave who embraced ART as means of increasing women's choices by offering control over their infertility. This agenda supported the commercialisation of the ART industry, which has seen it become an entirely legitimised medical practice that has thrived in the neoliberal context, but also significantly due to the exercising of choice by women to have children later in life.

Although largely an issue for wealthy countries of the global north, the availability of technologies to address infertility is also an issue of reproductive rights. As addressing infertility became a diverse, technologically assisted medical procedure that includes the purchase of harvested eggs (gametes), in vitro fertilisation, the use of donor eggs and sperm, a global market emerged. As noted by Schurr (2018) since the early success in 1978, a growing number of consumers have bolstered this market, those experiencing delayed childbearing, single people wishing to conceive, same-sex couples and heterosexual couples with infertility problems. Infertility treatments are available across the world and a competitive market means that people can shop around to find the best deal. According to Schurr (2018) four cycles of IVF could be purchased in the USA for $50,000, but that amount could cover ten cycles in Ukraine, surrogates could also be found there or in Mexico, and other places catering for 'reproductive tourists'. There are diverse regulations surrounding ARTs, as it is not only an unequal technology due to costs, but some countries or jurisdictions only permit such procedures for heteronormative married couples and not for unmarried or homosexual people.

In some countries, such as Australia there are government subsidies for ARTs, but the cost can still be prohibitive for low-income people. In Israel anyone, regardless of marital status, can access free fertility treatments, including IVF for two babies or until a woman turns 45 years of age (Kraft, 2011). This is seen as an effective and egalitarian policy in a country that places extremely high value on the notion of family and has one of the highest fertility rates in the world. In contrast, the Hungarian government announced free IVF in 2020 as part of the right-wing conservative, nationalist (anti-feminist) government policy that supported normative heterosexual families (lesbian couples and women over 45 years were excluded) as a measure to boost its population. Prime Minister Orban, who was re-elected in 2022, announced it as an anti-immigration policy and brought six fertility clinics under government control (BBC News, 2020). In a further policy aimed at rebuilding the native Hungarian population, he also announced very high tax incentives for women who had four or more children, a policy that only significantly benefits people who pay high taxes. Although these policies assist some people with the cost of a large family and some struggling with infertility, it is a very direct political exploitation of 'motherhood' to satisfy a racist anti-immigrant government policy. This is completely outside a social justice approach that would seek to reinforce reproductive rights for all, as these policies are being implemented in a context that has reduced social welfare overall and has high levels of poverty. In 2018, 16.2 per cent of the population of Hungary were in poverty (Juhász and Pap, 2018, p. 14). This invokes Corea's (1985) analysis that sees ARTs as 'medical mechanisms' for the social, medical, and legal control of women's bodies. It is not surprising then that Hungary is one amongst several countries in the European Union (including Poland, Austria,

Italy, Romania, Russia and Slovakia) that have low gender equality measures and are engaged in the backlash against 'gender ideology', which is directly in opposition to women's and girls' rights and women's representation in political power (Juhász and Pap, 2018).

In many cultures, the capacity to bear children is essential to a woman's cultural identity and is linked to the concept of fulfilment as a woman. Equally, it is argued that women should have a right to choose not to have children, but there are many accounts of how difficult it is for women who make that decision in heteronormative contexts. Tianhan Gui observed that Chinese and Japanese women choosing careers over the expected marriage and motherhood trajectory experienced social and family pressures and were seen as 'left-over' women in China and 'loser dogs' in Japan (2020, p. 1958–1959). Although it is difficult to argue that all families or individuals have a right to have children, it is equally difficult and socially unjust to deny access to technologies that equalise opportunities to have children. Reproductive technologies are commonly used for same-sex couples or for women and transgender men who do not have a heteronormative partner. Key welfare issues related to reproductive technologies are equal access, cost, medicalisation and in some instances, ethics.

In an argument for a new feminist perspective on issues of surrogacy and reproductive technologies, Holstrom-Smith (2021) explored a de-marketisation, anti-neoliberal approach. In promoting the broad idea of a strong welfare state and effective social welfare in relation to health and reproductive rights by outlining a reproductive justice policy agenda:

> Quality socialized medicine would address many common causes of infertility, while paid family leave would reduce pressures on women to delay childbearing. Reproductive technology such as IVF could be free for people's personal use as part of socialized healthcare. Barriers to adoption for LGBTQ couples and others who do not fit the white, nuclear, heteronormative family mould should be removed. Perhaps new models for raising children, such as non-romantic partnerships, could also be facilitated through changes to family law. Non-enforceable altruistic surrogacy agreements could potentially be a part of this diverse ecosystem of reproduction, enacting family formation as a type of mutual aid. In conclusion, activists and policymakers should work to create a public health and family policy that fosters the type of world we want to build. This world is inclusive, decommodified, and in which labor and love have priority over genetics and money. A reproductive justice policy agenda would have many facets, but commercial surrogacy would not be one of them.
>
> (Holmstrom-Smith, 2021, p. 484)

Given the now widespread use of ARTs, Holmstrom-Smith's (2021) vision provides a way forwards that embraces a reproductive justice goal, even though it does not overcome the global diversity of legal controls or impositions, lack of strong welfare states and economic inequalities that exclude many global South and some global North countries from adopting such an egalitarian approach. Like most feminist praxis in the contemporary world, the political and economic conditions and diversity of cultural contexts are barriers to a unified approach to reproductive rights.

Surrogacy

The phenomenon of surrogacy (where one woman is employed or volunteers to bear a child for another person or couple who can't have their own or for gay men wishing to have their own biological child) has prompted many debates since 1984 when it became a publicised issue in the infamous 'Baby M' case in the USA, when Mary Beth Whitehead agreed to be a surrogate for Elizabeth and William Stern. As the biological mother, she wanted to keep the baby but lost custody in a court of law. However, although a relatively recent feminist and social welfare issue, due to advances in reproductive technologies, it has become a common practice and led to debates about the commodification of women's bodies and the marketisation of children. Some feminists argue that it has also become a new layer of labour exploitation of women, particularly by the rich global North of women in the poorer global South. This can be seen as part of what Candace Johnson described as 'stratified reproduction', which is a term that 'conceptualizes the phenomenon that accords different values to reproductive tasks undertaken by women in different socioeconomic, cultural, and national contexts' (2017, p. 233). It particularly highlights the protected and respected place of 'reproduction and reproductive autonomy' for socially and economically privileged women and men of the global North when compared with poorer women or men within Northern countries and women in the global South (Johnson, 2017). This is obvious when in the USA, where in many states commercial surrogacy is legal, surrogacy arrangements cost between $90,000 to more than $200,000 and although more than 18,400 babies were born through gestational surrogacy in the USA, where the carrier is not related to the foe-tus, due to these high costs in the USA many potential parents sought cheaper options in countries like India and Thailand (Rudrapper, 2017). Clients for such services came mainly from the USA, Britain, Australia and Israel (all places where commercial surrogacy is illegal as it is across much of Europe) (Rudrap-per, 2017). In India it was estimated to be a billion-dollar industry, with 12,000 babies born in such arrangements, until 2018 when transnational and commercial surrogacy was prohibited across India and only available as a domestic, altruistic practice (Rozée et al., 2020). In their research, Rozée et al. (2020) interviewed 30 women who were surrogates in commercial operations and all of them saw it as an opportunity to address poverty or transform their economic status and felt positive about exercising their economic autonomy. India's withdrawal from this marketplace of course opened other sites for international surrogacy, includ-ing Ukraine and Mexico. Schurr (2018) pointed out the high level of disparity between young, white Western women with higher education who receive 100 times more for their eggs than sellers in India, Mexico, Ukraine or Georgia and a similar difference in compensation for being a surrogate in the global North and the global South.

In 2019, New York state, after banning commercial surrogacy in 1984, put forward a revised legislation to allow it, specifically due to pressure from gay male couples (Wang, 2019). Washington State and New Jersey legalised commercial surrogacy in 2018, joining about a dozen other states in the USA that had legalised it. More than 18,400 babies were born through gestational surrogacy between 1999 and 2014 in the USA, in cases where the surrogate was not related to the foetus. According to data from the Center for Disease Control and Prevention 10,000 surrogate's babies were born after 2010. There remain strong criticisms of and opposition to surrogacy, including a view that it is a form of 'reproductive prostitution'. Tatiana Patrone (2018) supported this view via a Kantian philosophical argument, which was derived from a position of moral judgement rather than feminist critique about exploitation. Surrogacy is compared to prostitution because commercial surrogacy enters the market, making women's bodies consumer goods because the women who become surrogates are not viewed as autonomous subjects or agents but as objects or commodities (Patrone, 2018). A Kantian philosophical perspective sees this type of commodification as morally impermissible. However, it is arguable that there is a clear distinction between surrogacy and prostitution in that the body of a surrogate is not *sold* in the same way as in prostitution. Kantian reasoning would argue that a person (or human) cannot or should not be used as a means and from a juridical perspective one cannot sell oneself into slavery. The one legitimate contract in which one can use their sex organs is marriage. Kant rejects the contract of prostitution due to its contrariness to morality (and in his view, reason). Patrone concludes that from a Kantian perspective '[r]egardless of one's motives, the practice that requires one to treat her body [or one's self] in a way that provides a service cannot be morally acceptable' (2018, p. 119). I have laboured over this somewhat as it explains, on the one hand, the inherently conservative nature of describing surrogacy as reproductive prostitution and to understand, to some extent, that it is a moral judgement. Patrone extends this argument further in the case of surrogacy, as, she argues, motherhood too cannot be divorced from gestation, 'because reproduction has to do with the use of not merely one's sexual organs but one's embodied self as a whole' (2018, p. 120). This latter position aligns more with feminist exploitation theories of surrogacy.

There are cases that highlight the exploitation critique of surrogacy and the inseparability of motherhood from gestation. For example, in Thailand, the law was changed to exclude international surrogacy after an Australian couple contracted a Thai surrogate that resulted in a successful twin pregnancy. However, the intended parents only took one child home and left the other child in Thailand. According to the surrogate mother, he boy twin was abandoned because he had Down's syndrome. The Australian couple claimed that the agency they used had only informed them of the one child, but as it had ceased as a business that claim was not confirmed. The surrogate mother kept the son and applied for custody of the daughter too. It was found that the Australian couple did not abandon the boy child. Later, however the father was imprisoned for child sex offences demonstrating a lack of duty of care in regulatory processes, which did not have the capacity to vet applicant parents for such contracts. Now surrogacy in Thailand is available only to heterosexual couples where one spouse is a Thai national and if they have been married for at least three years. Further, the surrogate must: be a sibling of one of the married couple; have had one child already; be married, and have permission from their husband. The new laws are based on morality about marriage and sexual identity in a country that outlaws but tolerates prostitution.

Like other ARTs, surrogacy has emerged as a globally marketised process that is here to stay, even though many countries have limited it to altruistic surrogacy, in which only a person close to the infertile couple can carry their child, for no commercial compensation, therefore excluding financial commodification and potential exploitation. This discussion has not focused on feminist practice in relation to ARTs, as it is a challenging and complex area of social welfare, but rather on where it fits, from feminist perspectives, in socially just welfare. It is possible that Holmstrom-Smith's (2021) proposition of all ARTs being made available to anyone who requires them through the socialisation of medicine, within a strong welfare state commitment, offers an acceptable place for surrogacy. As part of that vision, 'non-enforceable altruistic surrogacy agreements could potentially be a part of this diverse ecosystem of reproduction, enacting family formation as a type of mutual aid' (Holmstrom-Smith, 2021, p. 484). It is equal access to ARTs that can create a social justice approach within women's reproductive rights, however, due to the imbalance in wealth between the global North and the global South and between rich and poor communities within some of the richest countries in the world, equal access to any form of reproductive technology is a long way from reality.

Conclusion

As women's reproduction has been a focus of feminist theorising and activism for five decades, there have been significant emancipatory and cultural achievements for women's autonomy over their own bodies. However, what frustrates us, as resisters and as agents of social change is the lack of permanent, unassailable shifts in thinking and a widespread acknowledgment of women's agency over their own bodies. There continues to be many forms of societal, legislative and institutional control, forwards and back as governments move from progressive to regressive politics despite widespread support for a woman's right to choose. For example, attacks on the gains made for the right to choose to have an abortion are the most won and lost of such swings. Epitomised by contemporary politics in the USA after the Trump presidency, when state laws, run and controlled by staunch patriarchs, began reverting to stringent and punishing anti-choice legislation (Jacobs and Stevens, 2019), putting women's health and autonomy in jeopardy. In 2019 only nine out of 50 states in the USA had laws that protect the right to abortion (Jacobs and Stevens, 2019). Pro-life, conservative women and men, bolstered by their religious faith and righteousness, have reasserted an idea of womanhood as motherhood that is secondary to an unborn child. From this perspective, pregnant women are seen as vessels for producing a child, regardless of how a pregnancy occurred or their potential or capacity for being a parent. The wave of regressive changes in reproductive rights has met with strong feminist activism, in the form of public protests and legal action, but with the rise of authoritarian, populist governments across the world these rights are being systematically withdrawn in several countries. Rights to determine one's own reproductive experiences is also an area that has a sharp divide between global North and global South experiences, especially in relation to the nature of differing welfare states and the level of under-resourcing for women's health. Given the now historical success of women's movements in the global North in achieving recognition of specific reproductive needs, such as access to contraception, abortion, maternal health services and assisted reproduction, it is difficult to comprehend the extent to which the battles to gain such rights will have to be fought for again in some countries. For feminist practice in the field of reproductive rights, success lies in achieving widespread support in communities and across nations and continuing to assert the persistently troubling demand for gender equality.

References

ABC (Australian Broadcasting Corporation) (2019) Anti-abortion activists lose High Court challenge to laws banning protests outside clinics. *ABC News*, April 10, 2019. https://www.abc.net.au/news/2019-04-10/anti-abortion-protestors-lose-high-court-bid/10987714.

Alzate, M.M. (2009) The role of sexual and reproductive rights in social work practice. *Affilia*, 24 (2), 108–119.

arora, N. (2017) Menstruation in India: Ideology, politics, and capitalism. *Asian Journal of Women's Studies*, 23 (4), 528–537.

BBC News (2020) Hungary to provide free fertility treatment to boost population. *BBC News Online*, January 10. https://www.bbc.com/news/world-europe-51061499.

Bearak, J., Popinchalk, A., Ganatra, B., et al. (2020) Unintended pregnancy and abortion by income, region, and the legal status of abortion: Estimates from a comprehensive model for 1990–2019. *The Lancet*, 8 (9), E1152–E1161. https://doi.org/10.1016/S2214-109X(20)30315-6.

Bendavid, E., Boerma, T., Akseer, N., Langer, A., Malembaka, E.B., Okiro, E.A., Wise, P.H., Heft-Neal, S., Black, R.E., Bhutta, Z.A., Bhutta, Z., Black, R., Blanchet, K., Boerma, T., Gaffey, M., Langer, A., Spiegel, P., Waldman, R., and Wise, P. (2021) The effects of armed conflict on the health of women and children. *The Lancet (British Edition)*, 397 (10273), 522–532.

Caddick, A. (1995) Making babies, making sense: Reproductive technologies, postmodernity, and the ambiguities of feminism. In P. Komesaroff (ed.) *Troubled Bodies: Critical Perspectives on Postmodernism, Medical Ethics, and the Body*. Durham, NC: Duke University Press, 142–167.

Center for Reproductive Rights (2019) *The Tragic Impacts of Unsafe Abortion Care in Kenya Are All Too Real*. New York: Center for Reproductive Rights, January 24. https://www.reproductiverights.org/feature/wanjikus-story.

Corea, G. (1985) *The Mother Machine: From Artificial Insemination to Artificial Wombs*. New York: Harper and Row.

Daly, M. (1978) *Gyn/ecology: The Metaethics of Radical Feminism*. Boston, MA: Beacon Press.

Johnston-Robledo, I. and Chrisler, J.C. (2020) The menstrual mark: Menstruation as social stigma. In C. Bobel, I.T. Winkler, B. Fahs, et al. (eds) *The Palgrave Handbook of Critical Menstruation Studies* [Internet]. Singapore: Palgrave Macmillan. https://www.ncbi.nlm.nih.gov/books/NBK565611/#ch17.Sec3.

Good Bloody Period (2021) https://www.bloodygoodperiod.com/.

Grate, R. (2012) That time of the month: An excuse of sexism all the time. *The Representation Project Blog*. http://therepresentationproject.org/that-time-of-the-month-an-excuse-for-sexism-all-the-time/.

Gui, T. (2020) "Leftover women" or single by choice: Gender role negotiation of single professional women in contemporary China. *Journal of Family Issues*, 41 (11), 1956–1978.

Gunter, J. (2019) *The Vagina Bible: The Vulva and the Vagina--Separating the Myth from the Medicine*. New York: Citadel.

Her (2017) These are the most popular slang terms for being on your period. *Her* (Online magazine). (Accessed December 19, 2019). https://www.her.ie/life/these-are-the-most-popular-slang-terms-for-being-on-your-period-281136.

Hinsliff, G. (2021) There will be blood: Women on the shocking truth about periods and perimenopause. *The Guardian*, July 22. https://www.theguardian.com/society/2021/jul/22/there-will-be-blood-women-on-the-shocking-truth-about-periods-and-perimenopause.

Holmstrom-Smith, A. (2021) Free market feminism: Re-reconsidering surrogacy. *University of Pennsylvania Journal of Law and Social Change*, 24 (3), 443–484.

Im, E.-O. (2007) A feminist approach to research on menopausal symptom experience. *Family & Community Health*, 30 (1), S15–S23.

Jacobs, J., and Stevens, M. (2019) With abortion in the spotlight, states seek to pass new laws. *New York Times*, February 18. https://www.nytimes.com/2019/02/08/us/abortion-laws.html.

Johnson, C. (2017) Pregnant woman versus mosquito: A feminist epidemiology of Zika virus. *Journal of International Political Theory*, 13 (2), 233–250.

Johnson, B.R., Mishra, V., Lavelanet, A.F., Khosla, R. and Ganatra, B. (2017) A global database of abortion laws, policies, health standards and guidelines. *Perspectives*. World Health Organization (Updated June 2017). https://www.who.int/bulletin/volumes/95/7/17-197442/en/.

Juhász, B. and Pap, E. (2018) *Backlash in Gender Equality and Women's and Girls' Rights*. A study commissioned by European Parliament's Policy Department for Citizens' Rights and Constitutional Affairs (at the request of the FEMM Committee). https://www.europarl.europa.eu/RegData/etudes/STUD/2018/604955/IPOL_STU(2018)604955_EN.pdf.

Kelly, L. (2019) Irishwomen United, the Contraception Action Programme and the feminist campaign for free, safe and legal contraception in Ireland, c.1975–81. *Irish Historical Studies*, 43 (164), 269–297.

Kraft, D. (2011) Where families are prized, help is free. *New York Times*, July 17. https://www.nytimes.com/2011/07/18/world/middleeast/18israel.html.

Liminowicz, A. (2022) Declare it to a doctor, and it's over': Ukrainian women face harsh reality of Poland's abortion laws. *The Guardian*, May 10. https://www.theguardian.com/global-development/2022/may/10/ukrainian-women-face-harsh-reality-poland-abortion-laws?position=3.

Ndembi Ndembi, A.P., Mekuí, J., Pheterson, G. and Alblas, M. (2019) Midwives and post-abortion care in Gabon: "Things have really changed". *Health and Human Rights: An International Journal*, 21 (2), 145–155.

Nelson, J. (2019) Historicizing body knowledge: Women's liberation, self-help, and menstrual representation in the 1970s. *Frontiers (Boulder)*, 40 (1), 39–61.

O'Donnell, K.S. (2017) Reproducing Jane: Abortion stories and women's political histories. *Signs: Journal of Women in Culture and Society*, 43 (1), 77–96.

Patrone, T. (2018) Is paid surrogacy a form of reproductive prostitution? A Kantian perspective. *Cambridge Quarterly of Healthcare Ethics*, 27 (1), 109–122.

Plan International (2019) It's about bloody time: Tampons and pads should be free in Australian schools so no girl misses out. *Media Release*, May 27. Plan International. https://www.plan.org.au/media-centre/its-about-bloody-time-tampons-and-pads-should-be-free-in-australian-schools-so-no-girl-misses-out/.

Prendergast, C. (2018) How an abortion in 1910 changed the world, stories like that of Vera Connolly show how abortions change lives for the better. *Gen by Medium News Site*. https://gen.medium.com/how-an-abortion-in-1910-allowed-a-woman-to-change-the-world-f9fdc2a20647

Radnor, A. (2017) 'We're having menstrual liberation': How periods got woke. *The Guardian*, November 11. https://www.theguardian.com/society/2017/nov/11/periods-menstruation-liberation-women-activists-abigail-radnor.

Ranabhat, C., Kim, C., Aryal, A. and Doh, Y.A. (2015) Chhaupadi culture and reproductive health of women in Nepal. *Asia-Pacific Journal of Public Health*, 27 (7), 785–795.

Rozée, V., Unisa, S. and de La Rochebrochard, E. (2020) The social paradoxes of commercial surrogacy in developing countries: India before the new law of 2018. *BMC Women's Health* 20 (234) (Online). https://bmcwomenshealth.biomedcentral.com/articles/10.1186/s12905-020-01087-2.

Rudrapper, S. (2017) India outlawed commercial surrogacy – Clinics are finding loopholes. *The Conversation*, October 24. https://theconversation.com/india-outlawed-commercial-surrogacy-clinics-are-finding-loopholes-81784.

Sabban, Z.A., Patenaude, V., Tulandi, T. and Abenhaim, H.A. (2017) Obstetrical and perinatal morbidity and mortality among in-vitro fertilization pregnancies: A population-based study. *Archives of Gynecology and Obstetrics*, 296 (1), 107–113.

Safronova, V. (2019) Thousands of women have shared abortion stories with #YouKnowMe. *New York Times*, May 15. https://www.nytimes.com/2019/05/15/style/busy-philipps-abortion-youknowme.html.

Schurr, C. (2018) The baby business booms: Economic geographies of assisted reproduction. *Geography Compass*, 12 (e12359) (Wiley online library). https://doi.org/10.1111/gec3.12395.

Troutman, M., Rafique, S. and Plowden, T.C. (2020) Are higher unintended pregnancy rates among minorities a result of disparate access to contraception? *Contraception and Reproductive Medicine*, 5 (1), 16–16.

Utz, R.L. (2011) Like mother (not) like daughter: The social construction of menopause and aging. *Journal of Aging Studies*, 25 (2), 143–154.

Voicu, I. (2018) The social construction of menopause as disease: A literature review. *Journal of Comparative Research in Anthropology and Sociology*, 9 (2), 11–21.

Wang, V. (2019) Surrogate pregnancy battle pits progressives against feminists. *New York Times*, June 12. https://www.nytimes.com/2019/06/12/nyregion/surrogate-pregnancy-law-ny.html?searchResultPosition=1.

WHO (World Health Organization) (2019) *Contraception Evidence Brief.* https://apps.who.int/iris/bitstream/handle/10665/329884/WHO-RHR-19.18-eng.pdf?ua=1.

Wiseman, E. (2019) Jennifer Gunter: 'Women are being told lies about their bodies'. *The Guardian*, September 8. https://www.theguardian.com/lifeandstyle/2019/sep/08/jennifer-gunter-gynaecologist-womens-health-bodies-myths-and-medicine.

6

OLDER AND OLD WOMEN AND FEMINIST PRACTICE

Introduction

As every country in the world is experiencing the ageing of their populations, providing support and advocacy for old and very old citizens has become a major field of social welfare, social policy and welfare practice. This chapter focuses broadly on feminist analysis, social policy and feminist practice responses to the intersection between gender and older age. As noted by Toni Calasanti et al. (2006) and Charpentier et al. (2008), most feminist scholars have not given old age the attention it deserves, but when they have, they have focused on the processes and experiences of middle age for women, not the fourth, frail age. This results in a focus on ageing and ageism rather than the social and political status of very old women, and how sexism continues to affect their social welfare.

The principles and theorisation outlined here as feminist practice can and, it is argued, should be the framework adopted for working with all older people. As with other fields of feminist politics, advocacy and practice covered thus far in this book, practice in the field of ageing faces greater complexity with the intersection of ageing and other identities, geographies and experiences. However, for women entering old age, material, structural issues and identities such as their ethnic, racial, sexual, educational, parental, employment, health, dis/ability and relationship opportunities have already been bound up in and coloured by gendered expectations and restraints. This results in a high-level impact on their life course. Therefore, intersectional factors significantly determine the quality of the lived experiences of ageing, being older and being frail aged. Hence, this chapter explores key issues for older women and feminist engagement and practice in social welfare services or advocacy for older people. This includes the impact of ageism and sexism, heteronormative and institutional oppressions, and the historical, intergenerational impact of social, medical, economic and

DOI: 10.4324/9781315625188-6

employment practices and policies. Importantly, the chapter also examines how older women engage in feminist activism and social justice that aims to support older and frail aged people.

I argue that an emancipatory approach should frame social justice practice when working with older people. This approach is strongly aligned with the emergence and ongoing practice of feminism as the parallels between sexism and ageism are very strong and can be equally oppressive. Emancipatory practice, in this context, means to unequivocally resist and fight to free older people from the institutional, economic, social, legal and everyday ageist oppressions that they experience because they are older persons (Phillips, 2018). Taking this approach is not just about instigating freedom from ageist oppression, it is about supporting and creating opportunities for older people to continue to exercise their autonomy, agency and capacities to the fullest. Emancipatory practice is more than strengths-based or empowerment practice because of the indivisibility between supporting the agency of older people and working against ageism and other oppressive discourses about older age. Feminism has always been an emancipatory practice because it brings the battles of feminism against sexism and other gendered oppressions into advocacy, alliances and services as an indivisible purpose for action.

Although the generations of women moving into old and frail age are beginning to differ from the cohort who were constrained by the very conservative eras of reproductive and sexually aware adulthood prior to the 1960s, there are still many social constraints that were specific to women's life courses that have a resounding impact in their older age. This varies within different national contexts and cultures and from a life course perspective must be part of the personhood of each person who reaches older or frail age. But one common thread appears to be that experiencing growing older, and being old, is as highly gendered as the life course that led to becoming old.

As Browning et al. (2018) noted it is the gendered nature of education and employment and main care responsibilities that pose the most particular challenges in the pursuit of well-being in older age for women. This was demonstrated in a longitudinal study of trajectories of 'ageing-well' conducted in Australia over a 16-year period, as it found that women had zero probability of achieving a better 'ageing well' classification in later years, compared to men who had a one-in-five chance of improving their well-being in older age (Browning et al., 2018, p. 1). There is ample research that demonstrates in many areas of what has been broadly defined as social welfare in this book, where older women are and have been viewed and treated differently from their older male counterparts. However, it is the burden of the past 80 years' positioning of women in culture and society that has had the most profound, determining impact on how older women live out their older age. Recognition of the context of one's life course has gone hand in hand with women's struggles for equality and needs to be understood by contemporary feminists when seeking to engage and support older and frail aged women.

It is important to recognise that in today's world, not yet frail aged older women (between 65 and 80 years) face many challenges directly related to increased freedoms and rights achieved during or due to the second wave women's movement of the 1960s and 1970s in the many societies that have not completely transformed in the way feminists fighting struggles for equality had envisioned. This relates particularly to the enablement of women to divorce their husbands more easily or leave unhappy or violent relationships, to become sole parents or to be open about their sexuality and/or to choose independent or non-conventional, non-heteronormative lifestyles. Focusing on heteronormative family formations, according to the OECD Family Data Base (2020) marriage rates have dropped dramatically overall in OECD countries since the 1970s, but in some rich global North countries there have been increases in marriages, although they are happening much later in life. For example, in Sweden, the average age for women to marry is around 34 years, (OECD, 2020) a time in life when a person has had time to establish financial independence and some savings for retirement. The overall drop in marriage-rates, since the 1970s, has been accompanied by an increase in divorce rates, which seems to be related to relaxing divorce laws (OECD, 2020). For example, in Estonia, there were an unusually high number of divorces in 1995, most likely related to the introduction of a new family law that eased and simplified divorce procedures (OECD, 2020).

Such freedoms from patriarchal constructs earned by feminist activists were not necessarily accompanied by equally profound economic changes, attitudes to and support for the provision of care, educational and financial independence for women, nor improvements that resulted in equal pay or equal personal retirement savings. This mismatch in social change or failure of change to follow self-emancipated women into their older age, in many instances in the global North, has seen significant growth in homelessness and poverty for older women (AHRC, 2019; Phillips, 2017). The Australian Human Rights Commission found that there had been a 30 per cent increase in older women experiencing homelessness and that the dominant reason was escaping domestic violence, followed by housing crises and financial difficulties (AHRC, 2019). This experience is not exclusive to heteronormative women leaving husbands but includes transgender women, lesbians and women who have been single, living alone, have lost a partner or employment, suffering mental health issues, or have had poor educational opportunities (AHRC, 2020). In 2019, the gender pay gap was at 17 per cent in Australia, this lesser earning capacity and the common experience of having taken time out of the workforce for caring duties means many women cannot purchase their own home or even plan for the cost of retirement (AHRC, 2019). As noted by the AHRC about heteronormative women, immediately following a divorce:

> ...women generally experience a decrease in income (while men's income remains similar) and about 60% of women experience financial hardship

in the first year of divorce—unable to pay their mortgage or purchase essential items and reluctant to request financial assistance from friends or community organisations. Women are also more likely to lose home ownership than men and face multiple barriers when looking to buy other accommodation.

(2019, p. 13)

In global North contexts, widespread homelessness of older women is unprecedented in previous generations of women who had experienced more traditional marriages, or extended family care, that left them with some financial security due to their dependent spousal status, regardless of how difficult it may have been to remain in a marital home. Further, the failure of many societies and economies to recognise the labour of care has meant that primary carers in families, most often women, had limited capacity to prepare for financial, material security in their older age.

The specifically gendered nature of experiencing getting older, but still being of working age, and being in older and frail age is important in a wide range of welfare practices. A feminist lens brings into focus still pervasive gender inequalities that must be seen in the context of women's life courses, as each person has accumulated a personal history in either transformative or stagnant social, political and economic contexts. It is important to note that where women have had access to formal and informal education and political transformative social change towards greater equality, some older women have thrived both individually and collectively and have contributed widely to the welfare and advancement of others. It is also important to acknowledge that although this discussion focuses on older women, transgender women and men and other non-heteronormative people also face extreme disadvantage and often a burden of extreme prejudice as societies that may or may not have enabled openness of their identities as younger people, and systematically deny rights and opportunities for them as older people (Latham and Barrett, 2015). This can result in extreme loneliness and isolation after losing a partner and is particularly oppressive in an institutional care setting where heteronormative systems and prejudices prevail.

Highly influential in social policy and social welfare practice for older people, gerontology, a field of research concerned with ageing, old age and its attendant problems, often partnered with geriatric medicine, is a field that has gradually recognised and absorbed wider disciplinary perspectives. Most importantly, the field of critical gerontology includes contributions from feminist perspectives and theory linked to the early work of Simone de Beauvoir's (1972) *The Coming of Age* and more recent feminist gerontology scholars (Netting, 2011). Diana Garner encapsulated a feminist gerontological analysis of the positioning of older women in society:

We have systematically denigrated old women, kept them out of the mainstream of productive life, judged them primarily in terms of failing capacities and functions, and found them pitiful. We have put old women in nursing homes with absolutely no intellectual stimulation, isolated from human warmth and nurturing contact, then condemned them for their senility. We have impoverished, disrespected, and disregarded old women, and then dismissed them as inconsequential and uninteresting. We have made old women invisible so that we do not have to confront our patriarchal myths about what makes life valuable or dying painful.

(2000, p. 3)

I suggest the way older women have been isolated and marginalised relates not so much to 'patriarchal myths' but to deliberate historical exclusions and inequalities imposed by men to maintain power in both public and private spheres and, as Carroll Estes put it:

...the lived experiences and problems of older women are structurally conditioned rather than simply a product of individual behavior and choices. "Choices" and "preferences" (in economists' terms) that are available to women and other structurally disadvantaged groups are often highly constrained, if not illusory.

(2005, p. 552)

Older women are regarded in this way because they were mostly prevented from exercising their own capacity to take control of their own selves, burdened by traditional roles of caring, home management and supporting their spouse, ensured limited opportunities that support choices. We are in a time when women who were amid the feminist revolution of the second wave are becoming old and older. This chapter explores some of challenges to feminist social justice practice in working with older people. It also explores the question of how the feminist generation of older women are situated in society as ageing or older frail women and how they disrupt expectations of invisibility and passivity.

Global Perspectives on Ageing

The documentation of ageing from a global perspective largely relies on data about the ways and ages that people die, hence it is integrally linked to measures of longevity. Individual longevity depends on multiple factors of course, but as a statistic, it sets a benchmark for how long one can expect to live in a specific geographical and social context. Largely due to the success of improved health outcomes across most populations in the world, based on successful infectious disease eradication, improved medical interventions, services and treatments, improved workplace health and safety and some of the positive effects of globalisation in terms of access to food and nutrition, people are living longer. Although more recent research has seen a decline in longevity expectations in various countries around the world, including surprisingly the UK and the

USA where the lowest life expectancy is among women (Ho and Hendi, 2018), research in 2015 found that healthy life expectancy had increased in 191 of 195 countries. The increase of 6.1 years occurred between 1990 and 2015 (Kelland, 2016). However, the research also found that with the rise in chronological life expectancy, in general, people are also living more years with illness and disability. This has serious implications for the social welfare of older people and their access to sufficient resources to maintain a good life in their older age. In most countries, women outlive their male counterparts, making them the larger portion of the very old population. A 2017 Global Burden of Disease study found that globally, life expectancy was 73 years, but with a healthy life expectancy of only 63 years, meaning that on average ten years of life are spent in poor health (IHME, 2018, pp. 13–14). In addition, it was found that women experience a significantly higher likelihood of having a disability than men (IHME, 2018, p. 13) and as the primary bearers of children, the level of available maternal healthcare can also create long-term health deficits especially for women within low socioeconomic locations.

Given the examples above of drops in overall longevity in the UK and the USA, it is evident that the level of a country's wealth is a not a guarantee to of good health and well-being for older people. However, there are many global North countries that do have high life expectancies. Compared to the global average, Japan has the highest at 84.2 years, Switzerland at 83.8 years and Australia at 82.8 years (AIHW, 2020), which are examples of the highest life expectancy at birth, these countries have low relative poverty rates and strong social welfare that includes the widespread provision of healthcare, and secure retirement incomes. The USA has one of the highest infant mortality rates in the world, at 5.8 per 1,000 births, which affects the overall longevity rate (Cohen, 2021; Wallace et al., 2021). The recognised cause of the high rate of infant mortality in the USA is the failure in the provision of public healthcare as people from lower socio-economic groups are most likely to lose their infants (Cohen, 2021; Wallace et al., 2021). Research conducted by Wallace et al. concluded that 'improving health, reducing poverty, increasing reproductive rights, and expanding insurance coverage' (2021, p. 343) would be some immediate actions the government could take to address the infant mortality rate. The high level of poverty in the USA, for 37.2 million people (11.4 per cent of the population) (US Census Bureau, 2021) creates stress from the youngest to oldest members of its population. In 2020, the poverty rate was 16.1 per cent of people under 18 years and for people aged 65 and older, it was 9 per cent (US Census Bureau, 2021).

There is however significant regional variation in the experience of good or poor health in later years when different regions of the world are considered. This has a complex logic, as acknowledged above, unlike much 'disadvantage' it is not linked to overall wealth of a country or region as rich regions fare poorly in this group of statistics. Where women may be exposed to poor working conditions and poor access to education and welfare, they are more likely to spend their older age in poor health. For example, in South Asia, which includes Afghanistan, Pakistan, India, Bangladesh, Nepal, Bhutan and Sri Lanka, 92 per cent of women will live their extra four (only) years over the men in the region in poor health (IHME, 2018, p. 15). In contrast women in Eastern European countries who live 12 years longer than their male counterparts only 29 per cent experience poor health (IHME, 2018, p. 15). However, because 'lifestyle' diseases and causes of death accrue in wealthier regions, predicted poor health is relatively higher. In other words, in global North countries such as North America, populations of men and women had the worst healthy life expectancy at birth (Kelland, 2016). Rich country diseases such as 'diabetes, which is often linked to people being overweight or obese, and drug use disorders – particularly with opioids and cocaine – cause a disproportionate amount of ill health and early death in the United States' (Kelland, 2016). Moving beyond the health discourse, which dominates global perspectives on ageing, there are other observable gendered issues that highlight women's experiences of ageing.

From a global perspective, there is much research examining diverse cultural responses to caregiving for old people. This tends to reveal a high level of dependency on women as caregivers, both in the home and within institutional care settings. This often means a focus on cultural and gendered expectations of women within families to care for their older relatives. For example in a study of older Mexican immigrants in the USA, Jolicoeur et al. (2002) discerned differences between families who had acculturated (spoke English well, had longer term residence, etc.) and non-accultured families (preferred speaking Spanish and had lower paying jobs) this related to the cost burden to the women who were expected to and willing to take on the care duties and the differences of caring within the family home and external to it. What was similar between the different cohorts was the physical, emotional, and economic cost of caring for an older relative, but unacculturated women found extra stress from a general devaluation of old people in American society (Jolicoeur et al., 2002). This was seen in contrast to the value placed on old people in Mexico. The study also revealed that a lack of trust in American society led to a lower use of available support services that could lessen the burden on women carers. The overall findings related to the general lack of support by the state, owing to the low level of welfare state obligations to support old people and their carers.

Highlighting another common characteristic of older women's ageing experiences, in a study of older women in Singapore that explored leisure experiences, Peggy Teo (1997) found that the majority of grandmothers in the study were exploited for their reproductive labour by their children, relied on income transfers from relatives, lived in public housing, had no formal education, had been mostly homemakers or unskilled workers, lived with family members and their leisure consisted of extensions of reproductive labour and occurred mostly in the home. Teo noted the lack of formal welfare or social support that was available at the time and that 'the spatial bounds associated with gender roles and identities were reinforced by ageism' (1997, p. 666).

Ageism and Sexism: The Nexus of the Ageing Experience for Older Women

Ageism, it seems, is experienced by older people across the globe, even where we least expect it, for example in cultures that value elders differently to the commodified, capitalist global North (Teo, 1997). Recognised as the first researcher to analyse and name it, Robert Butler (1980) described three components of ageism, including prejudicial attitudes and beliefs about older people, acts of discriminating against older people and institutional policies that reinforce stereotyped notions of older age and result in a range of forms of individual and institutional oppression. Like sexism, ageism was only relatively recently recognised or even seen as a systematically imposed, dominant social view of older people. Also, like sexism, it is deeply embedded in Western, patriarchal, capitalist modes of production and consumption and relies on a dichotomous view between the high value of youth and youthfulness and the feared, lowly valued experience of getting older and of older age. As Laura Hurd Clarke observed:

> Sociocultural analyses of ageism have yielded profound insights into the structural inequities that precede and emanate from mandatory retirement policies, negative attitudes toward older workers, lack of access to health care and appropriate caregiving resources, and elder abuse.
>
> *(2010, p. 3)*

Chrisler et al. point out that 'weakness, frailty, passivity and dependence are also the aspects of the feminine gender role stereotype' that contributes to the intersection between ageism and sexism, reinforcing perceptions of older people as generally incompetent (2016, p. 89).

Dougherty et al. (2016) in an analysis of various studies about attitudes to ageing found that views of older women were distinct from those of older men as women were seen as largely asexual, less feminine than their younger counterparts, that their bodies should be hidden from view, and yet hyper-visible due to their failure to look beautiful. This barrage of negative perceptions can undermine older women's 'quality of life' because women often accept or subscribe to such cultural stereotypes and their loss of reproductive status can render women useless (Dougherty et al., 2016, p. 14). Rebecca Jones, in researching what an imagined feminist old age would be like, noted that there has been little social science research 'about the potential of feminism to enable ordinary people to reimagine old age', something beyond the current normativity of a neoliberal framework (2021, p. 1). In her study where she asked feminists to do that, it was found that people who identified as feminists 'generated ideas about a more inclusive positive old age' (Jones, 2021, p. 8). The imaginings, however, included mostly aspects promoted in the neoliberal context of independence, good physical and mental health, social connections and access to water for recreation, all contingent on a steady life course that enables a retirement income and capacity to live well. This indicates that it is difficult to break from an individualist, neo-liberal construction of what life should be like in older age, the subject of many government policies related to ageing and an enormous consumer market selling these ideas. The reality for many women across the globe is that their life course is disrupted by poverty, violence and/or loss or they have lived a life of secondary citizenship in a country where equal access to education and employment has limited capacity to facilitate independence in older age.

It is logical then that there are clear, specific consequences for the social welfare of older women due to the arrangements of economic, legal, and political structures that have either excluded or imposed vulnerabilities for older women through their gendered life course. However, one of the most intrusive barriers to being an equal citizen as an older woman is the overwhelming marketisation of the value of youth. The valorisation of staying young is based on intrinsic fears of getting old, which are the result of ageism. The commodification of youthfulness is omnipresent, it is a means of convincing people to use cosmetic surgery, to purchase 'beauty' products that are marketed as anti-ageing, to feel shame for looking old and to endure that getting old is circulated as both an insult and a joke. Such values are reinforced by mainstream media, by advertising and by the powerful music, television, and film industries as well as social media, which has a wide and influential reach. Although popular culture spheres are slowly changing (albeit to reinforce the separateness of older people as they make up a specific consumer market for old people being represented in media), the perfection of youth pervades the construction of what is beautiful and desirable. This also reaffirms a negative construction of ageing making it the opposite of what is beautiful. The intersection of sexism with ageism creates a double standard resulting in gendered ageism, that 'more severely and rapidly erodes women's than men's social valuation as they age' (Barrett and Naiman-Session, 2016, p. 764).

Although there are proponents of agelessness, viewing old age as a social construction, this is often placed on the older person to resist the category of old, the idea of ageing successfully or to be ageless, which is inherently ageist (Calasanti et al., 2006) and responsibilises the person to conform to ageist limitations about who they are. The idea of successfully ageing is thoughtfully analysed by Calasanti et al.:

> Successful aging requires maintenance of the activities popular among the middle-aged privileged with money and leisure time. Thus, staying fit, or at least appearing fit, is highly valued social capital. In this sense, successful aging means not aging, not being "old" or, at the very least, not looking old. The body has become central to identity and to aging, and the maintenance of its youthful appearance has become a lifelong project that requires increasing levels of work.
>
> *(2006)*

As further pointed out by Calasanti et al. (2006) a focus on and critique of age relations is essential for feminists to intervene in the oppressions that older people face. This is particularly important for people who are marginalised by difference or as they state 'intersections of multiple hierarchies' (Calasanti et al., 2006). For feminist practice with older people to be emancipatory, it must not only resist and challenge ageism but must also resist, acknowledge and challenge homophobia, racism and sexism. Such an approach would recognise that some older women, for example, enjoy privilege because they are white and heterosexual and are therefore treated differently to old black men, old lesbian women, and old transgender people. Ideas such as retirement leading to 'social solidarity in retirement' (Guillemard, 2002) add to the pressure for performing successful ageing and as Charpentier et al. point out adds to a risk of 'the marginalization and personal liability of sick and dependent old people who "haven't succeeded in aging well"'(2008, p. 346).

The nexus of ageism and sexism is, as mentioned above, an experience for women around the globe. The non-government organisation (NGO), HelpAge USA has a specific program for empowering older women, in which it intervenes to support women at risk of or experiencing ageism, violence and poverty. The following highlights these activities, demonstrating the universal presence of the ageism/sexism nexus and prejudice against older women:

> In Tanzania and other countries, witchcraft beliefs have led to an alarming number of witchcraft accusations. Anyone can make them, and they can be based on almost anything — like "bewitching" to cause illnesses. Allegations also come from family members who want control of a widow's property. The accused are usually vulnerable older women, and after being labeled as witches they are often brutally attacked or murdered. It's a complex issue that involves deep-rooted cultural beliefs, the low status of women, poverty, and other factors. Because of our interventions, there has been a 99% reduction in killings in regions where HelpAge and our partners have intervened.
>
> [For example]
>
> Fleeing violence and political turmoil in Burundi, Bernice settled into Tanzania's Mtendeli refugee camp. Soon after arriving she was accused of being a witch by the woman she was sharing a tent with — who wanted to coerce her into leaving so her boyfriend could move in. She told us: "I refused so they started spreading rumors that I am a witch, and that they don't want me in the village and that if I stayed, they would kill me. They came into my tent and beat me at about midnight."
>
> HelpAge's team in the camps helped Bernice move to a different zone in the camp away from her accusers and worked with the local communities to try to dispel myths about witchcraft.
>
> *(HelpAge USA, 2022)*

HelpAge USA works through an extensive global network across 80 countries that focuses on poverty and on the provision of social welfare, such as better health services, influencing government policies for better health care and specialised emergency assistance for older people. Although it is an organisation focused on older people in general, it recognises the specific conditions for older women, bringing a feminist perspective to its work.

Based on the experiences of ageism and sexism for older women, an emancipatory approach to the support and other welfare services for older people must also address the use of demeaning, infantilising language that circulates in wider society and particularly in institutional settings such as aged care homes and hospitals. Caldas-Coulthard and Moon (2020), in their study of discourses about grandmothers found that although references to individual grandmothers were often positive, a generic discourse about grandmothers was trivialising, derogatory, ageist and sexist. They also noted that contemporary grandmothers, women who have partners, are professional and continue to work, have not influenced widely circulating language about and perceptions of grandmothers (Caldas-Coulthard and Moon, 2020). Their analysis led to two key themes, social devaluation and gender bias, and found that in representations of grandmothers they were generally 'desexed', gendered only in the context of family, home and traditional 'female' pursuits (Caldas-Coulthard and Moon, 2020, p. 36). They found practices toward grandmothers resulted in exclusion and discrimination. This form of discrimination is based on ageist perspectives of older women in which they become invisible in the public sphere but are still exploited for their reproductive labour in the private sphere.

A more direct ageist language practice occurs in settings where feminist practice can directly intervene, in institutional settings. In such settings, older women are the focus of the business of those settings as women are the majority of very old patients or residents in hospitals or aged care facilities. The devaluing language used by professionals and other staff in these settings is often infantilising or dismissive, doctors appear to be the worst offenders in this respect according to numerous studies (Chrisler et al., 2016). Other studies have found that physicians and medical students have views that see old people as 'primarily related to death, disease, and decline in functionality' and stereotype them as 'rigid, religious, irritable, boring, lonely, isolated, asexual, easily confused, depressed and depressing, needy, frustrating, and non-productive' (Chrisler et al., 2016, p. 91). Chrisler et al. (2016) found that such attitudes were particularly marked in relation to older women and resulted in negative health outcomes for women as women can internalise stereotypical attitudes, resulting in weakness and dependency and unnecessary frailty leading to poorer treatment regimes in health settings. Chrisler et al. also noted that older women of colour have experienced a lifetime of racism, 'sexual minority women have long experience with homophobia, and transgender elders have experience with transphobia' (2016, p. 89). They also reported on a study by Sabik (2013) of African American and European American women in their 60s that showed how self-measures of their health related to perceptions of age discrimination and that the more discrimination they experienced the greater the impact on their physical health and mental well-being, not dissimilar to the impact on older lesbians who indicated frequent experiences of 'homophobia, heterosexism, and ageism in the healthcare system and elsewhere' (Chrisler et al., 2016, p. 89).

In institutional contexts, older women are often referred to as 'old dears', seen as cute or naughty if they protest or resist and often spoken to as if they were small children, not adults with a wealth of life experiences, knowledge, wisdom, and capacities. Chrisler et al. describe this as 'baby talk' where simple sentences with childish vocabulary are used, in a 'higher pitch and brighter tone' and for example, older women are addressed with terms like 'sweetie', 'dearie', and 'young lady' and by referring to a cooperative or compliant patient as a 'good girl' (2016, p. 93).

This kind of treatment in institutional care scenarios is tied to popular discourses about older women, as Caldas-Coulthard and Moon noted in reference to the power of the ideology of ageism:

> One of the consequences of the ideology of ageism is invisibility, silence, and stereotyping. Grandmothers and older people in general rarely have their voices heard in public spaces, but are represented in various derogative ways, … These stereotypes are ingrained in western societies and materialised in many types of discourse. Old women/grandmothers are referred to as "crones" or as "old bats" or "hags", or are othered for being old, weak, or dependent; postmenopausal women are positioned as mentally or physically deranged.
>
> *(2020, p. 39)*

An emancipatory practice would not only be conducted with a self-awareness of language use but would actively engage with others in the work context, to bring attention to the oppressive nature of language that belittles or infantilises. It would also involve appropriate and respectful engagement, building knowledge of the whole person and her life course, regardless of any illness or medicalised limitations. As discussed later in this chapter, in discussing care, institutional settings are driven by increasingly inhibiting neoliberal efficiencies that add an extra challenge to any form of emancipatory practice. A social justice feminist approach also includes pushing back against constraints on fulsome communication and engagement.

Older Women and Risk of Poverty

As discussed earlier in this chapter older women are at greater risk of poverty than men due to the many gender-based expectations and impositions throughout their life course. As noted by Carroll Estes, globally, women disproportionately suffer poverty and as a hallmark of old age, regardless of geographical location, and that 'the degree of dependency of older women on the state grows with ageing, widowhood, divorce, and associated declines in economic and health status' (2005, p. 553). Estes points to the impact of globalisation and neo-liberal pressures by institutions, such as the World Bank and the International Monetary Fund, place on governments to reduce expenditure and increase privatisation related to care, safety nets, financial support in retirement and health (i.e., the welfare state) that adversely affect older women around the world (Estes, 2005).

Research has shown that on a global scale, older women are more likely to live alone than older men, but the biggest factor is the lack of retirement income, United Nations research found that in 'the Asia-Pacific region, older persons, particularly older women, often rely on financial support from their families, but given that families are becoming smaller, younger generations will be less able to support their parents' (UNESCAP, 2019). Given the increasing number of women without children and never married the only means of avoiding poverty will be a form of 'secure access to both contributory and social pensions'. In the Pacific and South Asia, the system of age pensions is based on privatised individual contributions and for women who have had a lifetime of inequalities, with lower wages and/or interrupted careers, their accumulated contributions are significantly lower than men (UNESCAP, 2019), a situation duplicated across both the global North and the global South.

In South Africa older women are twice as likely to live alone than men and in Ethiopia, more older women than older men live alone (12 per cent of older women compared to 3 per cent of older men) (Samuels et al., 2018), many more women live with their children in the global South, where they are engaged in reproductive labour, caring for grandchildren, and doing housework. For women living alone, poverty is a higher risk, particularly in countries where there are weak or no welfare state or social protections. In the Samuels et al. (2018) research on older women in Ethiopia, it was evident that without the assistance of NGOs many women would not have basic social protections, including any form of income (Samuels et al., 2018). Although largely absent across the world, there are strong arguments for the inclusion of older women's security, support and economic status in macro as well as micro-economic policies (Samuels et al., 2018).

In one of the richest countries of the global North, USA-based research explored the question of whether US women still spent most of their lives married, which was a traditional status and informed most economic research's focus on households rather than women as a separate entity (Munnell et al., 2017). After examining 'four birth cohorts' from the early 1930s to the mid-1950s, they found that the years spent married had dropped from around 70 per cent for the older groups to 50 per cent for the mid-range baby boomers (Munnell et al., 2017). Their findings reflected an increasing number of women enjoying independence, based on three reasons, fewer women got married, getting married later and an increasing divorce rate (Munnell et al., 2017). As mentioned previously this kind of emancipation from patriarchal tradition had economic consequences for women as the world around them did not adjust to ensure gender equality in opportunities for work, education and economic security. The study found that the women in the study, nearly four in ten (39 per cent) women aged between 50 and 64, said the economy was 'not working well for them personally, compared to roughly three in ten women 65-plus, men 50–64 (33%), and men 65-plus (29%)' (Munnell et al., 2017). A majority were also worried about the cost of living, and nearly half of them said they had taken 'unplanned negative action' such as skipping medical care due to cost, prioritising a loved one's health, and skipping or reducing medication due to cost (Munnell et al., 2017). Highlighting the higher risk of poverty for women of whom half had become single in earlier years (50–64 years old), only nine per cent were confident that they would have enough money to live comfortably through their retirement years (Munnell et al., 2017). More of the older cohort, of whom 70 per cent were still married, were more confident (16 per cent) that they would have sufficient retirement income, although three times as many men felt they were likely to be financially secure in retirement (Munnell et al., 2017). This data supports the widespread understanding of increased vulnerability to poverty for older single women. Given this precarity and the high percentage of women living alone, one of the most profound aspects of being an older woman is the risk of not having secure housing.

Homelessness is one of the most obvious outcomes of poverty and research has indicated that the fastest growing group of people experiencing homelessness are older women, particularly in the 55 and over year-old group. This was supported by research conducted by the Australia Human Rights Commission, which found that women aged 55 and over were the fastest growing cohort of homeless Australians between 2011 and 2016, increasing by 31 per cent in that period and noted that the trend would continue, due to a 'shortage of affordable housing, the ageing population, and the significant gap in wealth accumulation between men and women across their lifetimes' (AHRC, 2019).

In Australia, in 2021 the majority of people using Social Housing Services due to becoming homeless were escaping domestic violence and of that group, 77 per cent were women (AIHW, 2021). However, it is unlikely that it captured the large number of older women, who are less likely to be visible or use generic social housing services. As noted by the Australian Human Rights Commission:

> Older women's homelessness is often hidden from view. Women experiencing homelessness often stay with friends or family, live in severely crowded dwellings, under the threat of violence or are physically hiding. In contrast, men often sleep rough, or live in improvised dwellings or boarding houses. Women additionally look to 'self-manage' their homelessness through strategies such as partnering up, moving between family and friends, and looking to take on jobs that provide housing.
>
> *(2019, p. 8)*

In a more recent detailed study in Australia, Debbie Faulkner and Laurence Lester (2020) found that around '240,000 women aged 55 or older and another 165,000 women aged 45–54' were at risk of homelessness. Their research pinpointed specific empirical characteristics that placed older women at a more likely risk of homelessness, which corresponded with facing risks of poverty. They included having been at risk before, not being employed full-time, being an immigrant from a non-English-speaking country, living in private rental housing, have difficulty raising emergency funds, being Indigenous, in a lone-person household or being a lone parent (Faulkner and Lester, 2020). An important response to the precarity of housing needs for older women was a demand for policy development to create affordable housing options for older women. A group called the Housing for the Aged Action Group (HAAG) embarked on a specific campaign to influence policy makers to develop an appropriate policy response that called for: an increase in the availability of affordable and appropriate housing for older women at risk of homelessness; investment in service systems to support older women before they reach a housing crisis; and addressing gender inequality in Australia (HAAG, 2020). Highlighting the broader problem of gender inequality demonstrates feminist practice, which included narratives from women's experiences of housing stress, the strategy was put forward in lobbying key political parties leading up to the 2022 election. There was a strong emphasis on older women's homelessness as a growing problem by highlighting that '400,000 Older Women Call for a National Housing Strategy' (HAAG, 2020). This discussion about housing for older women in Australia contrasts with countries where there is no system or policy of social housing (funded by government) but does demonstrate the risks for older women who also face forms of poverty, especially in countries where there are no or limited welfare state responses. In the Australian context, after nine years of conservative neoliberal governments, where women were not a priority social policy area and social housing had been largely privatised in most states, this high-risk cohort had been ignored, although some Labour government states had begun to address the needs of older homeless women.

An example of addressing the specific needs of older women's housing is represented in Melissa Fernandez Arrigoitia and Karen West's (2020) report on a study about a unique feminist co-housing project, established through the Older Women's Co-housing Network (OWCH), called New Ground, which after 18 years of battling 'institutional hurdles and societal ageism', was 'established in 2016 by a group of 26 women in the age range 52–89' in the UK (2020, p. 1673). The model, which relies on mutual aid among residents, is a means of older people 'ageing in place' instead of trying to sustain one's own home or going into some form of local, hard-to-find residential care accommodation (Arrigoitia and West, 2020). As an aged housing option it challenged the 'binary of 'independent' community dwelling and institutional provision' (Arrigoitia and West, 2020, p. 1674). The length of time it took to establish this form of housing was largely due to a lack of support from the building and development sector and local government, however, the women's activism and commitment saw it through.

Twenty-six women moved into the housing, and six of them had been member of OWCH for between 10 and 18 years, with support from possible future residents, who sometimes join outings organised by the residents (Arrigoitia and West, 2020). It is evident that this initiative emerged from a group of social justice-oriented activists committed also to a 'socially inclusive' ideal, so that women without housing equity and from diverse cultural, racial and sexuality backgrounds would also benefit from the housing model (Arrigoitia and West, 2020). This objective was enabled by partnering with other associations who could support them financially to have eight of the 25 dwellings established as a form of social housing (Arrigoitia and West, 2020). Arrigoitia and West noted that a 'further factor in hindering the establishment of a senior co-housing community was Britain's ageism and dominant paternalist culture towards the aged' as '[d]evelopers and housing associations appeared unable to listen to and work creatively with older people and particularly older women' (2020, p. 1674). This project is an ideal way for older women to live, given their diverse experiences and capacities for care and collaboration. Although there are other co-housing models it has the advantage of the concept of ageing in place, a clear desire for many old or frail aged people wanting to stay in their community. A key finding in Arrigoitia and West's research was the idea of the residents of the housing project 'embracing their housing future in a collective and agentic way [that] was not about "ageing successfully"', a problematic construction for ageing, as discussed earlier in this chapter, but about 'actually accepting their ageing selves as that process unfolds' (2020, p. 1691). The feminist framing of the New Ground, and OWCH, is representative of feminist practice that seeks to resist 'traditional patriarchal models of womanhood and ageing', particularly in how this form of alternative housing attempts to collectivise care work and challenges 'the gendered architecture of our lives' (Arrigoitia and West, 2020, p. 1692). The New Ground co-housing project reflects the activism and capacity of older women to plan and design for their own housing needs. As the residents articulated on their website:

> We are a group of women over fifty who have created our own community in a new, purpose-built block of flats in North London. As an alternative to living alone, we have friendly, helpful neighbours... We are carving out a path for other 50+ year-olds to follow. We hope they have an easier journey than ours, now we have shown the way. The senior cohousing community could enrich the lives of many, and reduce pressures on health and care services, if local authorities, planners, policy makers and housing developers helped to remove the many obstacles society puts in its way.
>
> *(New Ground Cohousing, 2018)*

As further noted on their website, in 2018, 3.64 million people over 65 lived alone in the UK and 70 per cent of that group were women. Addressing isolation and loneliness experienced by older people has significant health benefits, as research has shown that loneliness creates a 50 per cent increase in developing forms of dementia, premature death from all causes, increased risk of heart disease and an increase in hospitalisations, with older LGBTQI and immigrant elders at higher risk than the rest of the population (Centers for Disease Control and Prevention, 2021). Therefore, drawing on principles of collective feminist action for housing and care can reduce the high level of dependency on the state, which appears inevitable for older poorer women.

Care and Abuse

The gendered expectation of women to provide care throughout their life course is a central experience for most women in the world and has been a focus for feminist activists and researchers. The nexus between being a carer and requiring care in frail age is more likely to fall to women due to their longer life compared to men. However, many older men are also challenged by being old and having to provide care for their partner and in contexts where there are not sufficient social welfare services or family and community support, which creates risks of abuse, poverty, social exclusion, and stress. Some older and very old women are vulnerable to abuse in many of the same ways that women and others in intimate relationships experience domestic violence (UN, 2022). In the context of the family home, older people can be physically abused, emotionally controlled by coercive behaviour by other family members and, most commonly can suffer financial abuse by members in their family or community who 'care' for them. According to the United Nations (2022), financial abuse or exploitation, has been found to be higher among older women than among older men and that older women using care services, or who are divorced, separated, lonely, or isolated face increased risk of financial abuse. The private domain nature of this kind of abuse means that it has not been a visible social policy problem and therefore not a focus of advocacy or activism. As noted by Swedish researchers, Karin Johansson, Lena Borell and Lena Rosenberg an 'understanding of home tends to be based on romantic perspectives on the home as a place for safety, comfort and positive relationships, overlooking how the home can be an arena for conflict, discomfort and unsafety' (2022, p. 158). Therefore, for some older people the institutional setting of residential care is a better option for care, which makes nursing homes or residential care facilities important sites for emancipatory practice. In Sweden, where there is a strong welfare state that funds aged care in local governmental jurisdictions in situations that are a mix of private and non-profits residences, the overall quality of care is person centred (Johansson et al., 2022). In their study about how nursing homes created a sense of homeliness, Johansson et al. concluded that 'findings from this study illustrate how staff invited residents to be involved in everyday duties and to be a recourse for the shared everyday life at the nursing home' (2022, p. 175). Apart from demonstrating an overall emancipatory approach that recognised the importance of agency, their research demonstrated the positive importance of aged care as a social welfare issue, an issue for government resourcing and policy.

It has only been since the 1990s that there has been a growing global recognition of the occurrence and risks of abuse and neglect for older people and its elevation as a social policy or social welfare issue (Penhale, 2018). Elder abuse has been recognised by the World Health Organisation and the United Nations (UN) as well as NGOs such as the International Network of the Prevention of Elder Abuse. The UN reported:

> One out of six people aged 60 or over experienced some form of abuse in community settings in 2020, while two out of three employees in nursing homes and long-term care facilities admitted to having committed abuse against older persons in the same year …As the world continues to age, rates of elder abuse are expected to increase, translating to serious health, financial and social consequences to older persons and their communities. The intersecting forms of discrimination experienced by older women, coupled with their higher life expectancy, suggest that abuse and violence against older women is an issue of concern.
>
> *(2022, p. 4)*

As discussed above, institutional care is a site for the most visible oppressive ageist treatment for older people, especially women. In some countries, nursing homes and other aged care facilities have, under neoliberal governments, become less regulated, increasingly privatised and corporatised, the conditions for the increasing number of mostly women residents have become more vulnerable to low quality and even abusive care. The extremely high number of deaths due to the COVID-19 pandemic in aged care institutions in 2020, 2021 and 2022, reflected the low priority and poor health services that exist in many such facilities, specifically in global North countries such as the UK, Australia, Spain and the USA. In 2021 COVID-19 deaths were 41 per cent of all deaths measured across 22 countries, which was a lower rate that in 2020 (LTC Responses to COVID-19, 2020). A Royal Commission of inquiry into the highly privatised aged care system in Australia between 2018 and 2021 found an overall incompatibility between operational profit motives (such as lack of medical/nursing care and low staff/patient ratios) and high-quality care. In relation to abuse it found:

> The abuse of older people in residential care is far from uncommon. In 2019–20, residential aged care services reported 5718 allegations of assault under the mandatory reporting requirements of the Aged Care Act. A study conducted … for the Australian Department of Health estimated that, in the same year, a further 27,000 to 39,000 alleged assaults occurred that were exempt from mandatory reporting because they were resident-on-resident incidents. In our inquiry, we heard of physical and

sexual abuse that occurred at the hands of staff members, and of situations in which residential aged care providers did not protect residents from abuse by other residents. This is a disgrace and should be a source of national shame. ...Our analysis of abuse also focused on restrictive practices, which are activities or interventions, either physical or pharmacological, that restrict a person's free movement or ability to make decisions. Where this occurs without clear justification and clinical indication, we consider this to be abuse.

(Australian Government, 2021)

There were many poor outcomes for residents in aged care facilities during the pandemic crisis that must lead to better systems of institutional care, but the incidents of abuse indicated in the Australian government's Royal Commission Report were part of everyday events in institutions that had little regard for the agency or autonomy of residents. The failure of care found by the Royal Commission can be attributed to material limitations, where efficiencies to ensure maximum profitability, such as poorly trained and poorly paid staff, insufficient time spent with each resident to ensure proper care and overuse of medication as a form of control of 'difficult' residents, but license for these factors is an ageist disregard, that leads to views of older people as 'other', as somehow less human. This is a repeated positioning of oppressed groups in need of emancipation. This is the essence of the national shame named in the statement above and is why an emancipatory approach is required to free residents in many residential care institutions.

In terms of addressing the ongoing oppressive environment of the aged care institution, there have been some important innovations that have resulted in a progressive change toward a more emancipatory model of care (Phillips, 2018). Feminist practices facilitate this approach by recognising the specific experiences of women as the majority of people in frail aged care, and how their life course can inform practices that support their ongoing agency. This includes creating conditions that, even with patients suffering dementia, the identity and life experiences of residents are enabled to create a home-like environment rather than an institutional one. This also recognises the number of older women throughout the world who have high-level reproductive labour skills, with deep knowledge of how to care and how to manage and contribute to a home environment. It must also acknowledge the highly feminised workforce within aged care and recognise the value of their work by improving wages and conditions. An emancipatory approach for residents includes their active participation and influence in meals, opening access to kitchens, the recognition of personal friendship bonds among residents (for example, enabling people to attend the funerals of people they have known in the residence), drawing on skills and capacity of residents for group activities, ensuring information is readily available and clearly communicated, but more than anything recognising the high value of the labour of carers within the contexts of residences (Phillips, 2018).

One example of an emancipatory approach to institutional care is a nursing home in the Netherlands that houses university students in with older residents, the students get free accommodation in exchange for interacting with and teaching new skills to residents (such as computer and social media skills) (Harris, 2016). The benefits of such a program are that they challenge ageist stereotypes, address isolation and loneliness and contribute to a stronger sense of agency. The Netherlands has many innovative solutions to ensure that people in aged care enjoy a sense of home and belonging. A further example is the Hogeweyk Dementia Village. This enclosed facility creates an entirely familiar village context with a park, bars, and cafes, a supermarket, and a theatre, based on a concept that supports the agency of each individual resident. The Hogeweyk model seeks to address 'boredom, loneliness and hopelessness' and focusses on possibilities, not on disabilities', supported by trained professionals (DVA, 2022). This kind of innovation is part of a slowly emerging movement that recognises the oppressive nature of the traditional aged care facility. It is however a privilege of wealth in a country or a community that facilitates high-quality care. What is most important in activism that seeks to enhance the rights for all people to benefit from the recognition of agency, is for governments to take responsibility through subsidies and regulations that direct work towards transforming the nature of institutional care for old and frail people. A strong welfare state approach would ensure regulation against exploitation and abuse of the frail aged, as well supporting innovative models of care and the provision of subsidies for individuals with limited resources or incomes.

Feminist Practice by and for Older Women

Although much of this chapter has focused on the struggles and needs of older women, they are also a powerful resource for social change and social justice. The overwhelming proportion of volunteers in social welfare are older women and increasingly women, once past their 'mothering' and other care responsibilities, emerge as activists and leaders for change. Further, as noted by McHugh, from a USA perspective, the current generation of baby boomers includes the women who, have a past where they were leaders of marches 'for civil rights and women's rights, protested the war in Vietnam, and challenged sexual norms' (2012, p. 282). However, McHugh also noted that despite this wealth of activist political experience and a past that included higher education and work participation than the generations before them, they were largely not involved in activism (2012, p. 282). This broad generalisation is worth exploring, especially given the large number of studies located in Canada that highlight feminist activism among older women in contrast to McHugh's observation of older women in the USA. Charpentier et al. (2008) in exploring the activism of older women in Quebec frame retirement as an opportunity for involvement in political life as well as more engagement with family, friends, and community.

It is, however, important to consider why the women's movement has not been sustained by the women who were so central to it in the second wave, why this potentially powerful cohort of older women has been silenced. In her comprehensive narrative of the rise and fall of the women's movement in Peru, Celia Blondet (1995) described how the various threads of the movement, grassroots, militaristic and middle-class activists had come together by the late 1980s and achieved a great deal for women's participation in social welfare, by addressing human rights and poverty. However, she also describes how national economic reforms that lacked a social welfare program, left women's organisations to their fate of political fragmentation, poverty, and exclusion. By the 1990s, Blondet described the powerful impact of global neoliberalism:

> In Peru the power to regulate society has been given to the market, and the state has withdrawn its older social functions… The grassroots organisations, which played such an important role in providing a minimal safety net for the majority are in crisis and face the risk of complete isolation from the new forces facing the country today… Today the generally accepted discourse echoes the market and emphasizes personal initiative and individual growth and accumulation…Under these conditions, and in a context of poverty, violence, and neoliberalism the women movement(s) face an enormous challenge. A new scenario has emerged in which the state explicitly withdraws from its social function and leaves the market to order society.
>
> *(1995, pp. 271–273)*

In a further study of the Peruvian women's movement, particularly those involved in comedores populares, and their grassroots activities such as food kitchens providing meals for the poor that existed across Peru in the 1980s and 1990s, Moser (2004) challenged the idea of heterogeneity in the women's movement and described the complex impact of class differences. The insights she provided from the perspective of the grassroots activists demonstrated how middle-class academic feminists used the grassroots activists but excluded them from leadership in actions and failed to support their agency as feminists (Moser, 2004). Her insights are valuable as they can explain how many older women may be absent from feminist activism, having experienced this level of marginalisation. Moser (2004) further noted how failures of understanding among international NGOs also diminished the agency of grassroots activists by creating cleavages between the idea of a global feminism that is inclusive regardless of class and perceptions of activists in the global South. Based on the two separate historical examinations of the women's movement in Peru, it is evident that there are many factors that can inhibit women with previous histories as feminist activists to continue in their activism in older age.

Despite such barriers, there are many examples of older feminists engaged in activism and advocacy. One being a Canadian network, initiated by older women in 2011, called GRAN, which was mobilised in solidarity with grand-mothers from sub-Saharan Africa caring for their grandchildren whose parents had died of HIV/AIDS (Chazan and Baldwin, 2017). The leader of the group, 69-year-old, Sam, a retired feminist scholar, had focused on 'exerting pressure on the Canadian government and industry to adopt policies that would improve access to life-saving medicines, make schooling a priority for girls, and decrease the violence borne by women and girls throughout sub-Saharan Africa' (Chazan and Baldwin, 2017, p. 71). Chazan and Baldwin (2017) conducted a study of GRAN and its members, with the intent of enhancing an understanding of 'the complexity of contemporary feminist activism, especially in relation to the intri-cate roles and contributions of older activists' (2017, p. 74). Their wider interest was to add to the debate about the value and problems of the idea of feminist waves. In describing GRAN, the study showed that it was innovative as a wholly online organisation relying on an interactive website and online meetings and, later, engaging in social media (Chazan and Baldwin, 2017, pp. 75–76). It also used what might be seen as a second-wave feminist tactic of local consciousness raising and promoted the concept of 'grandmotherhood' as a pivotal discourse that created a non-threatening force for good (Chazan and Baldwin, 2017). Although the members of GRAN identified as feminists, they excluded that identity from the organisation's representation (Chazan and Baldwin, 2017) and based on its current website, there is no direct mention of feminism in its identity (GRAN, 2022).

An interesting finding of the study of GRAN members is that although they were of a similar age cohort that would fit the idea of the second wave, they had not necessarily been feminists in the 1960s or 1970s and many had come to feminism later in their life course (Chazan and Baldwin, 2017). An interesting analysis in Chazan and Baldwin's research findings was that the imposition of the feminist waves on older feminist activists was a form of ageism and 'that later life was a time of new and renewed activism for the women' in the research, which 'directly opposes any presumption that these women were withering away or disappearing from activist circles' (Chazan and Baldwin, 2017, p. 82). They also found that the members of GRAN engaged in their research stated that their activism went beyond the cause of women in Africa and functioned as a form of resistance to 'the invisibility and discrimination they experience in Canadian society as older women' (Chazan and Baldwin, 2017, p. 83). These findings reflect how feminist practice is applied as a political advocacy for agency as well as advocacy for improved welfare for communities that exist under poor or limited welfare states, as is the case in most African countries.

Conclusion

The aim of this chapter was to capture the diverse ways that feminist praxis and analysis can provide insights and activism that engages with the specific experi-ences of women as they become defined by their ageing and experiences of *being* old. Working from an emancipatory, social justice perspective with older people aligns with core principles of feminist practice, with a focus on agency, capacity and opportunity. It also requires resistance to and critique of ageism and sexism that is endemic to societal, institutional, governmental policy and human services contexts. The examples of feminist or feminist-aligned practice included in this chapter promote important perspectives that challenge sexist and ageist assumptions about older women and promote the capacity of collective action and emancipatory innovations in institutional contexts.

Although examples in this chapter are drawn mainly from global North data and responses, the specific risks of poverty and homelessness for older women are closely linked to the global experiences of losing relevance in cultures where the status of old people is not highly valued. Stereotypical, ageist and sexist views of older women often fix their value in reproductive labour, which is often exploited rather than valued as a set of skills that can contribute to environments such as, for example, residential aged care contexts. Alternately, most volunteers across social and human support and services are older women and their capacities for political action and policy influence are evident in contributions and leadership at local, national and international levels. Due to successful advances in societies that value and promote gender equality women have much greater educational opportunities, work careers and consequently building their saving to invest in their future retirement and older age income. For many women, their life course as carers and lack of access to education and secure work outside the home has meant they are destined to poverty in older age, especially if they find themselves living alone. A life course perspective is central to understanding trends such as the rapid increase in the number of women at risk of homelessness, possibly precipitated by intimate or domestic disruption, such as domestic violence or loss of a partner, but also affected by large contextual social, environmental (such as the COVID-19 pandemic) or economic changes. The other important context relates to the strength of social protection or social welfare provided by the state. The lack of a state-funded pension or regulated mechanisms for private retirement savings and the failure to have housing policies that support social housing and recognise the specific needs of older women place older women at greater risk. This is most important for older women because they live longer than their male counterparts and are more likely to spend their frail age with a disability, therefore they face a risk of poverty and dependency on available support from the state.

References

AHRC (Australian Human Rights Commission) (2019) *Older Women's Risk of Homelessness: Background Paper Exploring a Growing problem.* Sydney: AHRC. https://humanrights.gov.au/our-work/age-discrimination/publications/older-womens-risk-homelessness-background-paper-2019.

AIHW (Australian Institute of Health and Welfare) (2020) *International Health Data comparisons, 2020.* Canberra: Australian Government (Last updated October 20, 2020). https://www.aihw.gov.au/reports/international-comparisons/international-health-data-comparisons-2018/contents/life-expectancy-mortality-and-causes-of-death.

AIHW (Australian Institute of Health and Welfare) (2021) *Homelessness and Homelessness Services.* Canberra: Australian Government (Last updated December 6, 2021). https://www.aihw.gov.au/reports/australias-welfare/homelessness-and-homelessness-services.

Arrigoitia, M.F. and West, K. (2021) Interdependence, commitment, learning and love: The case of the United Kingdom's first older women's co-housing community. *Ageing & Society*, 41 (7), 1673–1696.

Australian Government (2021) Final report, executive summary. *Royal Commission into Aged Care Quality and Safety.* https://agedcare.royalcommission.gov.au/publications/final-report-executive-summary.

Barrett, A.E. and Naiman-Session, M. (2016) 'It's our turn to play': Performance of girlhood as a collective response to gendered ageism. *Ageing & Society*, 36, 764–784.

Blondet, C. (1995) Out of the kitchens and onto the streets: Women's activism in Peru. In A. Basu and C. McRoy (eds) *The Challenge of Local Feminisms* (1st ed.), 251–275. Ford Foundation, Women's Program Forum, Boulder: Westview Press.

Browning, C.J., Enticott, J.C., Thomas, S.A. and Kendig, H. (2018) Trajectories of ageing well among older Australians: A 16-year longitudinal study. *Ageing & Society*, 38 (8), 1581–1602.

Caldas-Coulthard, C. and Moon, R. (2020) The transgressive, the traditional sexist discourses of grandmothering and ageing. In C. Caldas-Coulthard (ed.) *Innovations and Challenges: Women, Language and Sexism.* London: Routledge, 34–59.

Butler, R.N. (1980) Ageism: A foreword. *Journal of Social Issues*, 36(2), 8–11.

Calasanti, T., Slevin, K.F. and King, N. (2006) Ageism and feminism: From 'et cetera' to center. *NWSA Journal*, 18 (1), 13–30.

Centers for Disease Control and Prevention (2021) *Loneliness and Social Isolation Linked to Serious Health Conditions.* Division of Population Health, National Center for Chronic Disease Prevention and Health Promotion (Updated April 19). https://www.cdc.gov/aging/publications/features/lonely-older-adults.html.

Charpentier, M., Quéniart, A. and Jacques, J. (2008) Activism among older women in Quebec, Canada: Changing the world after age 65. *Journal of Women & Aging*, 20 (3–4), 343–360.

Chazan, M. and Baldwin, M. (2016) Understanding the complexities of contemporary feminist activism. *Feminist Formations*, 28 (3), 70–94.

Chrisler, J., Barney, A. and Palatino, B. (2016) Ageism can be hazardous to women's health: Ageism, sexism, and stereotypes of older women in the healthcare system: Ageism can be hazardous to women's health. *Journal of Social Issues*, 72 (1), 86–104.

Cohen, J. (2021) U.S. maternal and infant mortality: More signs of public health neglect. *Forbes* (Online), August 1. https://www.forbes.com/sites/joshuacohen/2021/08/01/us-maternal-and-infant-mortality-more-signs-of-public-health-neglect/?sh=22a189553a50.

de Beauvoir, S. (1970) *The Coming of Age.* New York: W.W. Norton and Company.

Dougherty, E.N., Dorr, N. and Pulice, R. (2016) Assisting older women in combatting ageist stereotypes and improving attitudes toward aging. *Women & Therapy*, 39 (1–2), 12–34.

DVA (Dementia Village Associates) (2022) The Hogeweyk. https://hogeweyk.dementiavillage.com/.

Estes, C. (2005) Women, ageing and inequality: A feminist perspective. In Malcolm L. Johnson, Vern L. Bengtson, and Peter G. Coleman (eds) *The Cambridge Handbook of Age and Ageing*. New York: Cambridge University Press, 552–560.

Faulkner, D. and Lester, L. (2020) 400,000 women over 45 are at risk of homelessness in Australia. https://theconversation.com/400-000-women-over-45-are-at-risk-of-homelessness-in-australia-142906.

Garner, J.D. (2000) *Fundamentals of Feminist Gerontology*. New York: Routledge.

GRAN (2022) Grandmothers advocacy network. *About Us*. https://grandmothersadvocacy.org/about-us.

Guillemard, A.-M. (2002) De la retraite mort sociale à la retraite solidaire. *Gérontologie et sociétés*, 102, 53–66.

HAAG (Housing for the Aged Action Group) (2020) *Policy Snapshot, At Risk: 405,000 Older Women Risk Homelessness without Urgent Policy Reform*. Melbourne; Sydney: Housing for the Aged Action Group and Ventures Australia. https://www.oldertenants.org.au/sites/default/files/at_risk_policy_snapshot_and_key_findings_web.pdf.

Harris, J. (2016) Here's why some Dutch university students are living in nursing homes. *The Conversation*, November 29. https://theconversation.com/heres-why-some-dutch-university-students-are-living-in-nursing-homes-68253.

HelpAge USA (2022) Empowering older women. https://helpageusa.org/older-women/?gclid=Cj0KCQjw-JyUBhCuARIsANUqQ_JzUbrZKiQmBTQBv5EPJUsZpC92oalAAZRJmAB7tRRdueNrMWOHDowaAnzuEALw_wcB.

Ho, J.Y. and Hendi, A.S. (2018) Recent trends in life expectancy across high income countries: Retrospective observational study. *BMJ* (Online), 362, k2562.

Hurd Clarke, L. (2010) *Facing Age: Women Growing Older in Anti-Aging Culture*. Lanham, MD; Plymouth: Rowan & Littlefield.

IHME (Institute for Health Metrics and Evaluation) (2018) *Findings from the Global Burden of Disease Study 2017*. Seattle, WA: IHME.

Johansson, K., Borell, L. and Rosenberg, L. (2022) Qualities of the environment that support a sense of home and belonging in nursing homes for older people. *Ageing & Society*, 42 (1), 157–178.

Jolicoeur, P. and Madden, T. (2002) The good daughters: Acculturation and caregiving among Mexican-American women. *Journal of Aging Studies*, 16 (2), 107–120.

Jones, R.L. (2021) Imagining feminist old age: Moving beyond "successful" ageing? *Journal of Aging Studies*, 100950 (In press).

Kelland, K. (2016) Study shows health improving globally, but progress is patchy. *Reuters World News*. (Accessed March 12, 2018). https://www.reuters.com/article/us-health-disease-global/study-shows-health-improving-globally-but-progress-is-patchy-idUSKCN1260KX.

Latham, J. R and Barrett, C. (2015) *We're People First: An Evidence-Based Guide to Inclusive Services: Trans Health and Ageing*. Bundoora: La Trobe University.

LTC Responses to COVID-19 (2020) 2.00. Overview impacts of the Covid-19 pandemic on people who use and provide long-term care. *LTCcovid International Living Report on COVID-19 and Long-Term Care*. London School of Economics. https://ltccovid.org/international-living-report-covid-ltc/.

McHugh, M.C. (2012) Aging, agency, and activism: Older women as social change agents. *Women & Therapy*, 35 (3–4), 279–295.

Moser, A. (2004) Happy heterogeneity? Feminism, development, and the grassroots women's movement in Peru. *Feminist Studies*, 30 (1) (Spring 2004), 211–237.

Munnell, A.H., Sanzenbacher, G.T. and King, S.E. (2017) *Do Women Still Spend Most of Their Lives Married?* Center for Retirement Research, Boston College. https://crr.bc.edu/briefs/do-women-still-spend-most-of-their-lives-married/.

Netting, F.E. (2011) Bridging critical feminist gerontology and social work to interrogate the narrative on civic engagement. *Affilia*, 26 (3), 239–249.

New Ground Cohousing (2019) Welcome to new ground cohousing, a pioneering community for women. https://www.owch.org.uk/.

OECD (Organisation for Economic Co-operation and Development) (2020) SF3.1: Marriage and divorce rates. *OECD Family Data Base*. https://www.oecd.org/els/family/SF_3_1_Marriage_and_divorce_rates.pdf.

Penhale, B. (2018) Elder abuse, ageing and disability a critical discussion. In C. Bradbury-Jones and S. Shah (eds) *Disability, Gender and Violence over the Life Course : Global Perspectives and Human Rights Approaches* (1st ed.). New York: Routledge, 137–150.

Phillips, R. (2017) Women's poverty: Risks and experiences of poverty for Australian women. In K. Serr (ed.) *Thinking about Poverty* (4th ed.). Annandale: Federation Press, 137–147.

Phillips, R. (2018) Emancipatory social work with older people: Challenging students to overcome the limitations of ageism and institutional oppression. *Social Work and Policy Studies: Social Justice, Practice and Theory*, 1 (001). https://openjournals.library.sydney.edu.au/index.php/SWPS.

Sabik, N.J. (2015) Ageism and body esteem: Associations with psychological well-being among late middle-age African American women. *The Journals of Gerontology. Series B, Psychological Sciences and Social Sciences*, 70 (2), 191–201.

Samuels, F., Samman, E., Hunt, A., Rost, L and Plank, G. (2018) *Between Work and Care Older Women's Economic Empowerment*. London: Overseas Development Institute. https://cdn.odi.org/media/documents/12509.pdf.

Teo, P. (1997) Older women and leisure in Singapore. *Ageing & Society*, 17 (6), 649–672.

UN (United Nations) (2022) *Advocacy Brief Older Women: Inequality at the Intersection of Age and Gender*. United Nations Department of Economic and Social Affairs. https://www.un.org/development/desa/ageing/wp-content/uploads/sites/24/2022/03/UN-Advocacy-Brief-Older-Women.pdf.

UNESCAP (Unite Nations Economic and Social Commission for the Asia Pacific) (2019) Ensuring income security for older women in Asia-Pacific: Designing gender-responsive pension systems. *Social Developments Policy Brief, 2019/01*. https://www.unescap.org/sites/default/d8files/knowledge-products/SDPB%202019-01_Pensions%20Older%20Women.pdf.

United States Census Bureau (2021) *Income and Poverty in the United States: 2020*. United States Government. https://www.census.gov/library/publications/2021/demo/p60-273.html.

Wallace, L.A., Rucks, A.C., Ginter, P.M. and Katholi, C.R. (2021) Social factors and public policies associated with state infant mortality rates. *Women & Health*, 61 (4), 337–344.

7

FEMINIST PERSPECTIVES ON THE CRIMINAL JUSTICE SYSTEM AND THE LAW

Introduction

With a focus on broad social welfare implications, this chapter is a discussion of some of the various ways that the law and criminal justice systems are encountered, understood, imposed upon, negotiated and responded to by women and feminist practice. As a corollary to this, it is therefore unavoidable that there is also a focus on the ways that law and criminal justice systems, contain or even oppress groups of people and behaviours. Feminists have been long concerned about the gendered nature of the law and its manifestation in social policies and political and religious mandates. Feminists have also been concerned with how the law fails to promote and ensure gender equality, especially in countries that have transformed from colonisation or authoritarian regimes toward more democratic states and, in the process, have claimed principles of equality for all citizens. Unfortunately, the reverse is also occurring across the world, where hard fought for rights and legislative protections have and are being reversed, in countries that are turning back the clock because they have resumed authoritarian regimes or elected populist conservative governments. For example, in 2021, the Taliban took back the government of Afghanistan and despite its public pronouncements to modify strict laws for women it has resumed exclusions and controls that have forced women out of all public life, including leadership roles, legal and education roles and denying young women access to education and any form of social equality with men. This resulted in global feminist networks of women judges assisting women judges to escape who, along with their families, were in immediate danger (Cooper, 2022; Olivio, 2021) and women athletes assisting Afghan peers to flee their country (Wrack, 2021). This chapter will also discuss how women have intervened and changed laws as a form of feminist practice.

DOI: 10.4324/9781315625188-7

Feminist Practices in Challenging the Law

Changing laws or law reform striving for women's equal citizenship and equal treatment under the law have been widely important projects for feminist activists, lawyers, and welfare practitioners. In the global North, it was a primary focus of the liberal feminist agenda and central to early emancipatory movements. In the global South, women struggled to gain rights and abolish oppressive gendered practices supported by the law. For example, in both the 19th and 20th centuries in India there were localised women's reform movements fighting to improve the status of women and end oppressive, often legalised, practices that ensured women's second-class citizenship and, in many cases, direct harm (Bronitt and Misra, 2014).

Particularly due to the added impact of deeply patriarchal British colonisation and the connections between the suffragette struggle in the colonising country and colonised India, women fought for emancipation from colonial rule and both colonial and historical cultural patriarchal impositions. They also fought to repeal discriminatory laws and practices such as the requirement of dowries from a women's or girl's family when arranged to marry, the social exclusion or self-sacrifice inflicted on widows and the common practice of child marriage. Further, recognising that gender equality could only be achieved with equal access to representation, education and work, Indian women also demanded 'better education and equal political rights for women' (Bronitt and Misra, 2014, p. 38). Although a continuing practice in contemporary India, a Dowry Prohibition Act 1961 was achieved and later amended in 1984, which focused on legal responses to perpetrators of dowry-related crimes, including torture, murder, and rape (Bronitt and Misra, 2014, p. 38). Despite success in introducing early law reform, 'femicide' (the killing of women or girls because they are female) continues in contemporary India due to dowry costs (despite it being an illegal practice) and due to domestic violence, honour killings and stranger killings (Weil and Mitra vom Berg, 2016). Stranger killings in India are highly prevalent and relate very much to ongoing (although also illegal) caste-based hierarchical views of women and girls. According to 2016 research, 'non-intimate girl femicides include kidnapping for prostitution and trafficking, and rape of young girls followed by murder' are prevalent (Weil and Mitra vom Berg, 2016, p. 39). Girls from the traditionally lowest caste, Dalit, are common victims of rape and are often brutally murdered to shame and humiliate the lower-caste community, with very poor police responses to such crimes. The police response to such murders is 'selective with little outrage and high caste violators are shielded from prosecution' (Weil and Mitra vom Berg, 2016, p. 39). The targeting of lower caste women reflects an added vulnerability that poverty imposes on women. The lack of state welfare throughout India ensures that for many poorer people there is little protection from such vulnerability and little criminal justice for crimes committed against them.

A 2018 Thomson Reuters Survey found that India was the most dangerous country in the world for sexual violence against women (Bellinger, 2018), despite its significant economic growth and the rapid growth of a middle class. Such offences against women in contemporary India have significantly contributed to a widespread, vocal women's movement across the country. This movement has focused much of its energy towards improving rape and sexual assault laws and criticism of the failure of the judiciary to proceed with appropriate justice for women victims as, although in 2010 in the state of Tamil Nadu a 13-point plan to better protect sexual violence survivors was introduced by the Chief Minister who was a woman, only some of the initiatives had been introduced (Bellinger, 2018). At a national level, legislation on sexual assault in India does very little for victims of sexual assault. According to research conducted by Bellinger (2018), the low representation of women in the national government is a key factor in failing to legislate to protect women.

In the wider global South, citizenship gains have been achieved through legislative processes and challenges to the law, often by utilising external international frameworks such as human rights. However, more than a century after direct feminist calls for change, the right to be recognised as equal under the law is still a primary problem for women in many parts of the world. This relates to every sphere, including within societies in which women have managed to push forward and find more equality, but still face barriers that emerge from the generalised differences in gendered power. As noted by Atkins and Hoggett:

> ...the deficiencies [in the law] have almost always been those perceived by men from the point of view of a male-ordered world. Women's problems have become defined as problems because men have realized that if the law treated them in the same way as it treats women, men would consider it unjust. Thus, laws which seek to force women and men into separate spheres are now increasingly thought to be wrong, as are laws which put the stability of the home and family above the ordinary legal rights of the people within it. But there has been little enthusiasm for laws which seek to adjust the relationship between the separate spheres, to redefine what each entails.
>
> *(1984, p. 5)*

In other words, the historical legacy of law as an instrument of patriarchal societies has ensured that it has been designed by governments that have been dominated by men for centuries and in countries where feminism has not been a widespread social movement many laws remain stuck in that paradigm.

It is important to view the law through a feminist lens, a lens that asks just how equal women and marginalised gender groups are under the rule of laws, as it can often begin to explain gender disparities in everyday life. This is also related to how laws are upheld, policed, implemented, changed and protected. For laws to work effectively there must be policing and justice systems that function not only to support victims of crime but are available to challenge inequalities and discrimination and ensure fairness of treatment. For a fair justice system to function the principles and sentiments of laws must be followed. This requires a police force and judiciary that is led by social policies that inform laws that seek to protect everyone equally. It is at this juncture that the justice system appears most likely to fail to act without sexism, racism, classism and other prejudices, and there is a need to legalise positive discrimination in cases where inequality is deeply entrenched. For example, the extreme over-representation of minority groups across a population such as African Americans, Native Americans, Aboriginal Canadians, Indigenous Australians and many other First Nations Peoples in the respective justice and prison systems is one outcome of structural inequality and unequal justice. A just, human rights-oriented criminal justice system would embed a deep recognition and acknowledgement of the ongoing trauma and disruption caused by colonisation and develop laws appropriate to the historical legacies of colonisation and slavery.

Amongst such populations, women of colour are the most vulnerable and often invisible in the justice system. As noted by Gross, 'long-standing barriers to protection play central roles in the relationship among race, gender, violence against black women, and black female criminalization' (2015, p. 33). There are also important connections between Black American women having been subjected to domestic violence and sexual assault and their presence in the justice system:

> By 2011, when upward of 1 million women were either "incarcerated or otherwise under the control of the justice system," between 85 percent and 90 percent of those women reported a **history of** domestic and sexual violence as opposed to 22.3 percent of women nationally. Given black women's representation in the criminal justice system and their historic and ongoing vulnerability, there can be little doubt that gender violence is a key factor in their disproportionate representation. Indeed, 68 percent of incarcerated black women had been victimized by intimate-partner violence and compared to white women, black women are twice as likely to be killed by a spouse.
>
> *(Gross, 2015, p. 32)*

As is noted earlier in this book there are feminist activists working to assist mothers in prisons and as referred to later in this chapter, there are concerted efforts to address the specific conditions of women in prisons across the world. The intersection of race, gender identity and poverty are key factors for all prisoners and are aspects of identity that reduce the likelihood of fair or just treatment in the prison system.

Changes to Laws Affecting Women

Feminist activists and legal practitioners have achieved a great deal of reform in the law since the1980s, which due to the prevalence and influence of liberal feminism, has occurred most evidently in the global North. In Australia as in the UK, for example, laws related to rape were challenged and changed to include the full extent of sexual assaults that women had experienced, moving away from the singular definition of 'penile penetration' (Temkin, 2002, p. 55), and gender discrimination laws were introduced to prevent blatant gender-based discriminations in most spheres of public life. Certain aspects of the law took a great deal longer that others to change. For example, rape within marriage was still legal in some states in Australia until 1992, after being partially criminalised in South Australia in 1976 then, after NSW made it a criminal offence in 1981, other states gradually followed suit. As a public servant during the 1980s in the Western Australian government, I saw first-hand just how reluctant many men with institutional power were to adjust to significant changes in their worldview. This is because they saw mechanisms such as sex discrimination laws, positive discrimination, affirmative action or especially the introduction of quotas to seek better gender balance, as meaning they had to step back from their male privilege. When in fact such mechanisms were a means of achieving more equitable participation of women in decision-making, governance, and policy design. However, three decades later, there remain strong echoes of this reluctance. For example, on International Women's Day in 2019, the Australian Prime Minister, Scott Morrison stated that 'We want to see women rise. But we don't want to see women rise only on the basis of others doing worse' (Karp, 2019). In this statement, 'others' are, by default, men.

Under conservative governments, antifeminist sentiments drive both social and economic policy decisions and, if they have the power to do so, conservative governments try to turn back the clock and undo the gains that feminists and the women's movement made during the 1980s and 1990s in transforming laws and forms of equal justice. This is a worldwide phenomenon as populist conservative leaders are elected. In the Republic of Korea, a country with the lowest female work-participation rate and highest wages gap for women in the OECD, a new president was elected in 2022. Yoon Suk-yeol, campaigned vowing to abolish the government's gender equality ministry with anti-feminist rhetoric and claims that South Korea's low fertility rate was linked to increased gender equality, 60 per cent of men in their 20s voted for him (Rashid, 2022; Shin, 2022).

As mentioned in the previous chapter the backlash against women's rights had been brought into sharp focus in the USA under President Trump and the equally populist and conservative President Bolsonaro in Brazil, as for example, laws allowing women access to legal abortions are being dismantled. Also, although not successful at banning abortions completely, Viktor Orbán, Hungary's far-right populist prime minister, exemplified the backlash against women's rights by offering funds for major hospitals to stop performing abortions (Hungarian Spectrum, 2017), banning the teaching of gender studies, offering tax-free status for women who have four or more children, legislating the so-called 'slave law' that allows employers to demand unlimited amounts of overtime and not have to pay for it for up to three months, which largely affects unskilled female workers (Walker, 2018). Under the Orbán government, female representation in politics has been very low and has gone backwards since 1990 and is at the worst level in a list of 28 European Union nations when it comes to gender equality (Walker, 2018). It is critically important for feminist activists to recognise and acknowledge that the ideology of governments will determine how much effort goes into using the law to ensure women's equality and how much is required to reform and advance laws that are women friendly and support women's equality.

In countries that have gone through major transitions from colonial or authoritarian regimes to democratic governance, women have often been equal players in resistance, revolution or mass demands for freedom and major reform, but do not end up with an equal benefit from the transition. A case in point is South Africa, where, according to research conducted by Catherine Albertyn (2011), due to the race-based rather than gender-based redistributive polices and laws in the post-apartheid state, economic inequalities have kept poor black women at the bottom of the socio-economic hierarchy. She observed that 'South Africa was and remains a deeply patriarchal society in which women have been subordinated to men in public and private life' (Albertyn, 2011, p. 3). She further stated that although there were successful gender equal adjustments in the post-apartheid constitution providing 'potentially transformative standards for law reform', which addressed many 'traditionist' and cultural gender inequalities, poverty remains the biggest barrier for many black women to gain equality. She also noted that more recently 'male-traditionalists have (re)gained power, requiring women to defend equality rights in relation to decision making (political) power within traditional communities and access to land, a key resource in the traditional rural economy' (Albertyn, 2011, p. 155).

Transformations in the law and the status of women under the law appear to lag a long way behind societal transformations. It is always surprising to consider how recent legislating against domestic violence has been in many democratic countries. For example:

> In Korea, two pieces of domestic violence legislation were introduced in 1997: the Special Act on Domestic Violence (referred to as the "Punishment Act"), and the Prevention of Domestic Violence and Victim Protection Act ("Protection Act"). Once the 'Punishment Act' and the 'Protection Act' were enacted, the government, police, prosecutors' office, courts, counselling centers and various types of shelters for victims all worked together to put these laws into practice. However, the rate of domestic violence has not decreased. Rather, it has increased. This is not because domestic violence itself has increased but because women no longer tolerate male violence and are more likely to report it to the police.
>
> *(UN, 2007, p. 2)*

In Japan it was not until 2007 that a law was introduced to protect women against spousal violence, the president of Kenya launched the National Policy on Prevention and Response to gender-based Violence in 2014, a law against violence against women was introduced in Argentina in 2012 (UN Women, 2016) and in South Africa, a law against rape in marriage was introduced in 1993 (Albertyn, 2011). In many countries, women were also seen as a problem when they married and were legally forced to resign if they got married while employed in a range of professions such as public servants, teachers, or nurses. Even though the 'marriage bar' for public servants was abolished in 1946 in the UK, it was in place in Australia until 1966 (Sawer, 2016) and for teachers' and nurses' marriage bars were lifted by different states over the next four years, up to 1970. In the USA all marriage bars ceased in all professions with the passing of the Civil Rights Act in 1964. Despite these reforms toward 'improved' equality nearly 60 years ago, it was still necessary to introduce sex discrimination laws in the 1980s and even now women earn less than men for the same work across the world.

The World Bank reported in 2019 on how women's employment and entry into business in 187 economies were affected by legal gender discrimination, and determined an average national performance score of 74.71, indicating that a typical economy gives women only three-quarters of the legal rights of men. It also found that 'the average score in the Middle East and North Africa is 47.37, meaning the typical economy in that region gives women less than half the legal rights of men in the measured areas' (World Bank, 2019). It did find that there are six economies that now provide equal legal status for women in employment and business: 'Belgium, Denmark, France, Latvia, Luxembourg, and Sweden, all of which scored 100 in the Women, Business and the Law index, meaning they give women and men equal legal rights in the measured areas. A decade ago, none of these economies scored 100, indicating they had all instituted reforms over the past ten years' (World Bank, 2019, p. 2). The World Bank research looked at legal and regulatory measures that supported factors such as women's upward mobility in private sector workplaces, legal access to childcare, impact of marriage, pay equality, access to finance and assets, property and inheritance and retirement incomes (World Bank, 2019, p. 4). This research demonstrates that across the board women have had to seek reforms in every aspect of equal workplace participation and many countries still have a long way to go using the law as a mechanism for equality. Being able to work is directly related to social welfare as it provides the major means of social security. This is particularly the case in countries with weak or no welfare provisions and is increasingly so under advanced neoliberal economies where work is seen as the best form of welfare.

There is ample evidence that the law lags in gaining equality for women in many areas, but the law is also often hostile to women seeking to use the law to protect themselves or to *seek justice* through the legal system. Although at the 'lower' end of degrees of sexual assault, sexual harassment is illegal, and has been the focus of contemporary young (fourth wave?) feminist action, including the emergence of the #MeToo movement. Even though #MeToo began as a grass-roots movement driven by women tired of sexual harassment and assault, it rose to high levels of publicity when celebrities revealed experiences of harassment and sexual assault by powerful men in the film industry in the USA. It is evident that if women feel supported in reporting such assaults, they will proceed in very public ways and, in at least some cases, prosecution of the offenders followed. For example:

> On October 5, 2017, the New York Times broke the Harvey Weinstein story. High profile actresses including Ashley Judd and Rose McGowan accused Weinstein of propositioning and assaulting them while pursuing acting roles. In years past, Weinstein enjoyed a high level of power and prominence as a Hollywood kingmaker …The Weinstein story kept growing as additional stars described similar experiences. Weinstein was fired by his own company on October 8, 2017, which later declared bankruptcy. He has since been arrested on rape charges.
>
> *(Tippett, 2018, p. 230)*

The global growth of the movement was facilitated through social media when in 2017, actress Alyssa Milano requested that Twitter followers respond to her Tweets with the hashtag Metoo, identifying as victims of sexual harassment or sexual assault. This resulted in the Metoo hashtag being used on more that 12 million occasions (Tippett, 2018). However, as Tippett (2018) noted 'although Milano's tweet brought global attention to the MeToo movement, it originated from activist Tarana Burke. Burke started the movement in 2007 and used the term "metoo" to express solidarity with girls and women who experienced sexual assault' (2018, p. 231). This process demonstrated the effectiveness of establishing a place for women and girls to speak from, an important 'empowerment' process that brought focus on men's sexual and predatory violence and poor behaviour towards women. In the USA, where the high profiles cases emerged and were pursued, Tippett (2018) claimed that it has had an impact on how workplace harassment allegations and procedures are now followed up. Rather than the focus being on the failure of employers' policies, the focus shifted towards the acts and impact of harassment. Tippett wrote:

> The MeToo movement, particularly when combined with shifts in judicial interpretations and legal reforms, stands to have a lasting effect on employer disciplinary practices. Employers are likely to continue to take a more punitive approach to documented harassment. A more punitive approach will encompass a broader range of meaningful discipline than termination alone, and will likely include demotions, promotion denials, pay cuts, or other loss of status. Employers are also likely to alter executive employment contracts and privacy policies to provide themselves with more latitude to discipline employees for documented harassment, and to disclose those decisions if necessary.
>
> *(2018, p. 236)*

Although the #MeToo movement appears to have had a significant, widespread impact on the response to workplace harassment in the USA, Tippett did warn that the use of tweets to reveal harassment may be currently protected by a progressive (political appointments under the Obama administration) National Labor Relations Act Board (NLRAB) but new appointments by the Trump regime could mean that the positive effects could be fleeting (2018, pp. 151–152). This is a further example of how the law can work for women but can be wound back by conservative politics that tends towards unfettered freedom for men's actions, often trivialising women's complaints.

Where the Law Fails Women

It is a generalised experience for women and others (including men, transgender, non-binary and queer people) across the world that if they are raped or sexually assaulted, they will not necessarily achieve any form of justice despite being a victim of a crime and a violent personal violation. Here I will focus on women, as the achievements in the law and practice gained by feminists tend to create opportunities for others to see justice also. Demonstrating the failure of criminal justice and the ongoing denial of consent to sex as a human right, in 49 countries in the world (mostly Muslim or other strongly religious states) there are still laws that explicitly allow women to be raped in marriage, which reflects wider attitudes to men's rights and privileges over women within the law. In some of those countries, more recent domestic violence laws may afford protection to some women and some laws that explicitly deny that a woman can be raped in marriage, make exceptions for girls in child marriages. This is the case in India for example, where in 2022, despite an ardent struggle by Indian feminists to have the laws reformed. As noted by activist Mariam Dhawale, General Secretary of the All India Democratic Women's Association (an organisation that operated across 26 states and had 9 million members as of 2022), which had filed a petition to the High Court:

> After marriage, it's the husband's right over the body of the wife, and this concept that a woman can refuse sex within marriage is not widely accepted...In fact, it was not even accepted by the government. That's why the exception continues today.
>
> *(Frayer, 2022)*

As reported in the 2019–2021 National Family Health Survey of 724,115 women, conducted by the Indian government, around 30 per cent of Indian women aged 18–49 reported having experienced spousal violence and that the average Indian woman is 17 times more likely to be sexually violated by her husband than by anyone else (Ministry of Health and Family Welfare, 2021).

As mentioned earlier in this chapter, laws that now protect women from rape in marriage are relatively recent in many countries. Notably occurring because of feminist action within the women's movement such changes took place beginning in the 1970s but also as recently as the early 1990s when many laws related to sexual assault were reformed (Temkin, 2002). Despite the introduction of such laws in the 1970s, Temkin provided an account of how widespread marital rape was in the UK nearly 20 years later:

> …Kate Painter's thorough and comprehensive quantitative study of marital rape in Britain, conducted in 1989, may now be said to provide the final answer to those who have argued that marital rape is a rare event in this country. Out of a representative sample of 1,007 married women, it was found that 14 per cent or one in seven had been raped by their husbands. Painter points out that 'if this finding is generalised to all married women aged between 18 and 54, it means that over one and a quarter million (1,370,000) women who are or have been married have been raped by their husbands'. In almost half of the rapes violence was threatened or used. One in five women were pregnant at the time. Half of the wives raped with violence had been raped six times or more. The study echoes previous findings in revealing that marital rape was the commonest form of rape. In the survey it was seven times more common than rape by a stranger and twice as common as rape by acquaintances or boyfriends. Social class and geography were found to be significant. Wife rape was higher among women lower down the social scale, …Wives who were economically independent were found to be no less vulnerable to rape. The highest reported incidence of marital rape occurred amongst those who were separated or divorced at the time of the survey. Fifty-nine per cent of all those in the survey who had been threatened and raped and 51 per cent of those who had been hit and raped during their marriage were divorced or separated.
>
> *(Temkin, 2002, pp. 74–74)*

Evidence from this study supports a well-known view that rape, in general, is a highly unreported crime across the world. In a substantial national study in the USA, it was found that although one in seven women indicated having been raped in their lifetime, reporting of rape was around 16 per cent for that group (Wolitzky-Taylor et al., 2011). The barriers to reporting appear to have remained unchanged for decades, seen as a witness-less crime, fear of being blamed, of not being believed, shame, risk of further persecution, public exposure in the court system and risks of being attacked again. This includes appalling treatment by police who perpetuate the false rape myth of women falsely reporting rape in their own interests (Temkin, 2002). Feminist activists and practitioners in support services for women victims of rape or sexual assault have and continue to be in an uphill battle in this area.

At its essence, in incidences of rape or sexual assault, there is often a misconstruction of the idea of consent and, worse, that somehow men when driven by sexual desire or domination are entitled to force sexual encounters. It is still a prevalent view that men cannot really be held responsible for their actions when sexually aroused, as demonstrated in a 2017 national survey on 'Attitudes Towards Violence against Women and Gender Equality' conducted in Australia, the survey found, on the statement that 'rape results from men not being able to control their need for sex', 33 per cent of the those surveyed agreed (Webster et al., 2018, p. 7). The research concluded in its analysis of data related to consent, there was evidence of a denial

> of the requirement for sexual relations to be based on the presence and ongoing negotiation of consent. These attitudes rationalise men's failure to actively gain consent as a 'natural' aspect of masculinity (e.g. that women are passive in sexual matters).
>
> *(Webster et al., 2018, p. 11)*

A further statement that was agreed to by 42 per cent of respondents was 'it is common for sexual assault accusations to be used as a way of getting back at men' (Webster et al., 2018, p. 12). Such findings in the survey are endemic of a failure in the feminist project to completely erase the notion of women's secondary status in interpersonal and institutional relations and is a way of understanding the challenges faced in the welfare of women who have been raped and are not able to be protected or defended in the justice system. Efforts to include affirmative consent in criminal law have had success in some jurisdictions, in 2022 the government of New South Wales (Australia) announced a requirement for consent to be asked for and agreed to in every sexual encounter (Lang, 2022). The legislation had been passed six months earlier, but an adjustment period was seen as necessary for police and courts to adjust their approach to rape cases and was launched with a public education campaign about the meaning of consent. The new affirmative consent laws were the result of decades of advocacy by feminist sexual assault support organisations and the advocacy efforts of one young woman, Saxon Mullins, who had experienced sexual assault and after going through a trial saw the attacker released based on the ambiguity around consent in the law (Cormack, 2021).

There are of course many ways feminist practice had sought to address the failure of justice for sexual assault, and the reluctance of women to report it or engage with police or the justice system due to the hostility of that system. Feminists in the 1970s had to fight to have rape taken seriously by police and it was due to the efforts of a Chicago activist, Marty Goddard, the inventor of the rape kit to be used to collect evidence in hospitals when a rape victim presented, that police had the capacity to use it as forensic evidence, thus facilitating rape being recognised as a crime (Kennedy, 2020). However, as reported by Pagan Kennedy when she uncovered Ms Goddard as the real inventor of the kit:

> I was infuriated when I read a few years ago about the hundreds of thousands of unexamined rape kits piled up in warehouses around the country [USA]. I had the same question that many did: How many rapists were

walking free because this evidence had gone ignored? Take for example, the case of Nathan Ford, who sexually assaulted a woman in 1995. Although a rape kit was submitted to the police, it went untested for 17 years. During that time, he went on to assault 21 other people, before being convicted in 2006.

(2020)

Despite the facilitation of pursuing sexual assault as a criminal offence through changes to the law and the collection of forensic evidence, police and the justice system mostly fail to act in favour of sexual assault survivors. It was reported that between 2010 and 2017, more than 140,000 sexual assaults were reported to Australian police but around 12,000 of those reports were rejected by police because they did not believe a sexual assault had occurred (Ting et al., 2020). Of the 34,000 cases 'cleared' by police without making an arrest, more than half were withdrawn by the survivor and of the remainder only 30 per cent led to any legal action (Ting et al., 2020). The extreme variation in the number of sexual assaults reported to and rejected by police across different jurisdictions in Australia reflects the common experience of women and girls not being believed by police (Ting et al., 2020). In research from around the world, this is a very common experience for women, and it reflects a deeply entrenched idea that women invite sexual advances from men because of how they dress or where they go or are lying to get revenge. What is most troubling about these widely perpetuated views is that they reflect a deep-seated sense of male privilege to use women for sex, an idea most transparent in the fact that still, in many countries, the law views a man forcing sex on his wife as acceptable and that consent is not a factor for consideration.

Feminist responses to this fundamental affront to women's social welfare include widespread protest, establishing support services and engaging young women and girls in awareness of predatory behaviour, but most importantly of their right to be free of the fear of sexual assault and to be able to report it. One example of using social media to address at least one aspect of this is a service established by an Australian sexual assault service. The South-Eastern Centre against Sexual Assault established an anonymous reporting, mobile-friendly website called SARA (SARA, 2019). The purpose of the service is to provide an opportunity for women to break their silence about the assault anonymously. As a result of finding a way to speak of it around half of the women using the site then decide to report the assault to the police or at least attend sexual assault counselling. As Germaine Greer (2018) suggested, in her controversial commentary on rape, this process allows the victim to take over her narrative and become a survivor.

Abortion and the Law

For feminist practice it is important to recognise how controlling or policing women's bodies is central to maintaining an unequal status for women. As discussed in Chapter 5 of this book, the right to a safe abortion is one of feminism's most fought for legal rights for women. It is based on the long history of women having to take desperate measures to control their own fertility when faced with an unplanned pregnancy. In countries that had or have restrictive laws against abortion, women face risky procedures that lead to injury or death. For example, in the Philippines, where abortion has been totally banned for over century, one thousand women die per year from unsafe abortions (Aspinwall, 2019). Debates about 'pro-choice' (the right for women to choose to terminate a pregnancy) and 'pro-life' (the denial of woman's rights over the rights of an unborn foetus) relate also to the dominance of patriarchal views of women's rights in general and is manifested in religious institutions asserting moral power over legislative decisions by governments. In general, populations (in Australia and the USA, for example[1]) support the right to choose, even if they would not personally have an abortion or like the idea of an abortion. This indicates that, in a democracy, the laws in this area relate much more to women's autonomy than the effect of laws on limiting the number of abortions. It is an area fraught with risk and consequence, girls or women can be a victim of violence, rape or incest and become pregnant, then suffer institutional violence by being disallowed from terminating that pregnancy and, under different institutional circumstances, being forced to give up a child for adoption. Also, many women seek to terminate pregnancies due to poverty, because they cannot afford to have and raise a child. These factors ensure that regardless of access to legal safe abortion women will take risks with unsafe abortions.

In the English-speaking world, we hear constant reference to the threat to the Row versus Wade legal decision in the USA, which was a 1973 decision in the Supreme Court that passed a constitutional amendment to protect women's right to privacy and within that, a right to reasonable access to abortion, effectively legalising abortion (Bernadi et al., 2012; Reagan, 1997). However, a detailed history of the challenges that arose immediately after that decision, seen as a retreat from the assertion of a basic right, mostly brought about by states pursing their own restrictive legislation on abortion, reveals the ongoing desire for control over girls and women's bodies. Measured against constitutional rights to privacy and autonomy many challenges took place through case law that saw a toing and froing between restricting and supporting women's autonomy. This included decisions about parental consent or parental notification for minors, husbands' consent to their wives procuring an abortion, and periods of pregnancy that required different engagement with medical decisions (Gabrielson and Milender, 2013). Nicole Ratelle (2018) pointed out that the decision has continued to become more unstable, never allowing absolute autonomy in decisions to terminate a pregnancy and has affected more contemporary access to medication abortion, which has led to criminalisation of self-managed abortion. Ratelle provided an example of this form of criminalisation:

> Idaho resident Jennie McCormak was arrested and charged for the use of abortion medication to successfully terminate her pregnancy. McCormack

lived 140 miles away from the nearest abortion clinic in Salt Lake City, Utah. When she found out she was pregnant despite using birth control, she already had three children, no income other than some child support and no car. Since Utah had a mandatory seventy-two hour waiting period, having an abortion at a clinic would have meant two trips to the clinic and would have cost between $400 and $2000 depending on the gestational period of the fetus. ...McCormak got enough money to buy $200 "abortion pills" prescribed by an online provider. Two months later McCormak received the pills in the mail. Although her pregnancy was farther along than recommended for medication abortion, McCormak successfully terminated her pregnancy.

(Ratelle, 2018, p. 206)

After telling a neighbour who reported her, McCormak was arrested and charged with a felony violation, as it turned out there was insufficient evidence for a conviction and charges were dismissed (Ratelle, 2018, p. 206). However, the narrative of this women's needs and action for her own and her children's welfare in a situation of poverty, provides insight into the value of the autonomous use of medication abortion. Ratelle (2018) argued that simply allowing people to conduct their own medical abortion in the privacy of their own home is not just a matter of the law but is directly related to how the state supports overall social welfare. She cites the fact that only 14 per cent of workers in the USA had access to parental leave in 2016 and noted the precarious nature of safety net (basic welfare) funding as such limitations 'can determine the social, civic and economic role a person will be able to hold in society' (Ratelle, 2018, p. 211). In other words, access to the capacity to exercise the autonomy or to have a true right to a medication abortion is a social justice issue that is linked to the role and interests of the state in social welfare. Further, a positive right to abortion would see funds or free medical services made available to poor people to exercise that right. Ratelle framed this issue as a reproductive right, 'based on the idea that people should be able to decide if, when and how to have children and to raise them' (2018, p. 213).

At the time of writing this book, there had been a tide of changes in state legislation outlawing abortion across Republican states in the USA, taking advantage of the judicial appointments made under the conservative Christian-influenced Trump regime, in the hope to overturn the Roe versus Wade constitutional amendment. These moves have been extreme, for example the Alabama Senate approved laws making abortion illegal from the moment of conception, with no exceptions for victims of rape or incest and for anyone caught performing an abortion, they would receive a 99-year prison sentence (Valenti, 2019). As noted by feminist columnist, Jessica Valenti:

...It will be the most extreme anti-abortion law in the nation, voted into effect by men who had trouble articulating the most basic facts about women's biology, conception, or even how the law itself would function.

When Senator Clyde Chambliss, a Republican, for example, was asked if the law would allow for incest victims to obtain abortions, he responded: "Yes, until she knows she's pregnant."

He did not elaborate on how someone would have an abortion before she knows she's pregnant, outside of claiming, "It takes time for all the chromosomes to come together".

(2019)

Due to the federal law that supports rights to women's reasonable access to abortion, many state governments in the USA have legislated to impede access to safe abortion through restrictive requirements on medical centres that provide abortions, this is called Targeted Regulation of Abortion Providers (TRAP Laws). For example, requiring corridors wide enough for two gurneys to pass, expensive staffing requirements and requiring the centres to be a certain distance from schools.

These excessive and unnecessary government regulations – an ever-growing trend among state legislatures – increase the cost and scarcity of abortion services, harming women's health and inhibiting their reproductive choices. These laws jeopardise women's access to safe, legal, high-quality reproductive health care and represent a backdoor attempt by politicians to end legal abortion access. They are typically enacted based on the false pretext of protecting women's health and safety but have a clear ulterior motive of making it more difficult to provide abortion services and thus more difficult for women to obtain such services. For example, at the time Governor Phil Bryant signed Mississippi's Admitting Privileges Bill into law in 2012, he declared 'Today you see the first step in a movement to… try and end abortion in Mississippi' (Center for Reproductive Rights, 2015).

The point of highlighting these obstructions is to demonstrate the lengths that pro-choice politicians will go to deny women's autonomy. It is also an important welfare issue for poor women, women who cannot afford to travel interstate, or to Mexico, to find a clinic, the same women who cannot afford to have another or any child.

As a former U.S. colony, Philippine law criminalises anyone having or assisting in an abortion with sentences of six years (Aspinwall, 2019). It has been reported by the UN that bans on abortion harms poor women and other disadvantaged groups and that 'the average maternal mortality ratio was three times greater in countries with restrictive abortion policies in 2013 (223 maternal deaths per 100,000 live births)' than in countries with access to abortion policies (77 maternal deaths per 100,000 live births) (United Nations, 2014, pp. 14–16). In practice, abortion is allowed in cases where the pregnant person's life is at risk, but no law explicitly states this.

As the USA is one of the largest funders of official foreign aid, the impact of their anti-abortion policies had widespread ramifications for feminist practice supporting women's reproductive freedom and autonomy in the global South due to the 'Mexico City Policy' or 'Global Gag Rule', which Trump reinstated in 2017 (Brice and Wroughton, 2019; Russell, 2019; Starrs, 2017). Under this policy foreign nongovernmental organisations (NGOs) that received U.S. aid for family planning programs, were required to certify the non-provision of abortions, abortion advice, counselling, referrals, or advocacy for the liberalisation of their country's abortion laws ('even if they use non-US government funds for these activities') (Starrs, 2017). The consequences of such policy impositions have led to increases in abortion rates, as a key aspect of family planning clinics is to also offer and educate about contraception, therefore this policy has led to reduced use of contraception and closures of family planning health clinics (Brice and Wroughton, 2019: Starrs, 2017). The rule also potentially raised the risk of maternal deaths and endangered children's health worldwide. The USA also announced that it would expand the policy, by restricting NGOs from funding other NGOs that support abortion (Brice and Wroughton, 2019). In 2021 the newly appointed USA President Biden, rescinded the Gag Rule, 'as part of a series of executive orders aimed to improve access to affordable health care in the U.S. and around the world' (Center for Reproductive Rights, 2021).

The reintroduction (as it had been put in place by several Republican administrations for 34 years previously) of the Global Gag Rule elicited a global response, for example a coalition of more than 130 organisations endorsed the following statement, 'Supporters of global health and development, women's rights, gender equality, and free speech oppose the harmful global gag rule and reject efforts to undermine the health and rights of women around the world' (Bingenheimer and Skuster, 2017). A program called 'She Decides' funded by the Dutch Ministry of Foreign Affairs was established to counter the impact of the rule and '357 world leaders issued a high-level statement', which asserted that 'the Global Gag Rule would reverse decades of progress on reproductive, maternal and child health by putting critical health and family planning services and supplies out of reach for those who most need them' (Bingenheimer and Skuster, 2017, p. 280). Apart from diminishing the capacity for grassroots and international NGOs to provide safe abortions, prevent unwanted pregnancies, improve women's health in general and reduce maternal mortality rates, the Gag Rule also affected countries' capacity to meet their international obligations (Bingenheimer and Skuster, 2017). This included failure to comply with international human rights to recognise that the denial of access to safe abortion is a denial of basic human rights as it is integral to a woman's right to 'health and life' as well as slowing progress towards key Sustainable development Goals (SDGs) (Bingenheimer and Skuster, 2017). The SDGs, which the USA had signed up to, are goals that seek to address maternal mortality, women's health and well-being and gender equality, these goals for services are affected if services are constrained by policies such as the Global Gag Rule. This is a critical issue for understanding feminist practice as it demonstrates the extent to which men in power can curtail support for women's autonomy. Of course, this rule and all legislative changes being made by

Republican states in the USA by pro-life (or pro-foetus) lawmakers prompted widespread protest and commentary by feminist activists.

By focussing on the USA in this discussion, the aim was to highlight how gendered power can be exercised through lawmakers and how their ideology and legislative power sets out to limit women's autonomy. Pro-life activists ignore intersectional factors that lead women to needing abortions, and don't take actions such as supporting access to contraception, education of men to behave more responsibly, campaign against rape or incest or address widespread poverty. The wider issue of abortion law is indicative of a central, ongoing struggle within feminist practice as the implications of not having access to legal safe abortion is not simply about denying a service to women, it is a core social justice issue that results in adversely affecting poor women to a significantly greater extent. Prohibitive laws mean that poor women who live in countries or states that have made abortion illegal or inaccessible are at risk of or suffer, as discussed in detail in Chapter 5 of this book. Common negative experiences on women's social welfare are why the deeply political struggle to legalise access to safe abortions is a central issue for feminist practice, it touches all aspects of social welfare for women and girls as well as the fundamental issue of the right to reproductive autonomy.

Despite regressive turns in abortion policy in the USA, Latin America, during the same period, has undergone what has been termed the Green Wave. The Green Wave, due to intense activism by feminists in a broad-based women's movement across several nations, including Argentina, Mexico and Colombia, has brought about significant legislative changes to decriminalise abortion. In relation to Mexico:

> We know that there is not a specific profile of the person who undergoes an abortion, but there *is* one of those who are criminalized for doing so: women living in poverty, women of color, and those already living on the outskirts of society. But this is over [with the recent ruling]. The judgment passed by the Supreme Court fully recognizes, at last, that abortion is a right, not a crime.
>
> *(Global Fund for Women, 2022)*

However, this is not the case in all South American countries. For example, abortion is still criminalised in Brazil and in Honduras where laws remain that do not allow the sale of the morning after pill, which gives wide access to women and girls to terminate or prevent an unwanted pregnancy. Feminists across the world are involved in campaigns to bring pressure on governments to address this. One such campaign is via AVAAZ, which called for support in the following way:

> Hundreds of girls and women are raped and forced into motherhood every year in Honduras, while being denied fundamental rights, like emergency

contraception. Although the first ever female president can change this with just one signature, she's under heavy pressure to give up! Join the global call to let her know we have her back and expect her to deliver on women's rights.

(2022)

The campaign collected more than 700,000 signatures to include in a petition to be delivered to the new president. This action is an example of using social media for the gain of reproductive rights.

As Sommer and Forman-Rabinovici (2019) point out the struggle for reproductive rights, especially abortion, is integral to the global struggle for gender equality and it involves key spheres of action: the nation-state; civil society (faith-based organisations in particular) and intergovernmental organisations. They note World Health Organisation data calculates that there around 56 million abortions carried out each year and that every seven maternal deaths are as a result of unsafe abortions (Sommer and Forman-Rabinovici, 2019). This demonstrates not only the unevenness of abortion access across the world, but deadly costs to this limitation on women's rights. Although the process of gaining legal abortion relies on various spheres of action and activism, it is only a nation's laws and social welfare policies that ensure certainty for women's autonomy over their bodies and choices.

Women in the Prison System

Research indicates that even though women make up a relatively small proportion of prisoners across the world, there has been dramatic rise in the number of women imprisoned in recent decades (Jeffries, 2014; Jeffries and Newbold, 2015; Kajstura, 2019). This has been particularly pronounced in the global north and the phenomenon is directly related to social welfare issues. During the 1980s and 1990s, there was an increasing punitiveness and expansion of the criminal justice system, and simultaneous retrenchment of the welfare system in austerity trends across many global North states toward 'work as welfare' reform. This trend resulted in a decline in welfare provisions, especially in the UK, Australia and the USA, whilst imprisonment rates increased substantially.

Feminist practice also recognises the risks imposed on transgender women when placed in men's prisons. Through a study conducted in men's prisons in New South Wales (NSW) (the state with the largest prison population in Australia) Wilson et al. (2017) found that in addition to some extreme examples of rape, transwomen were subjected to continual sexual harassment and their sexuality was under constant negotiation. Their research concluded that although transwomen found ways of surviving men's prisons, they were much safer in women's prisons (Wilson et al., 2017). In NSW the law allowed transgender people to choose which gendered prison they wanted to go to in most cases and this was found to be an appropriate policy for transwomen going into the prison system.

According to Penal Reform International (2021) over 700,000 women and girls worldwide were either serving a sentence or awaiting trial, reflecting a 17 per cent increase since 2010 and that their specific needs are routinely over-looked. They also reported that a key reason for the increased number is that in some countries harsher approaches are being taken toward women committing offences in contexts of 'violence, coercion, poverty or discrimination' (Penal Reform International, 2021). Further, in some countries, such as Afghanistan or Saudi Arabia and Uganda, women are being imprisoned for 'status offences', including specific behaviours, such as feminist political participation/activism, using social media, adultery, sexual misconduct or prostitution (Penal Reform International, 2021).

In a large study conducted by Heimer et al. (2012) results showed a direct relationship between poverty and geographical concentration of African American communities and black women's imprisonment rates, whereas non-black women's imprisonment rates were unaffected by a growth in poverty. Another telling statistic from the USA, was that 62 per cent of women in prison had yet to be convicted and:

> ...the number of unconvicted women stuck in jail is surely not because courts are considering women to be a flight risk, particularly when they are generally the primary caregivers of children. The far more likely answer is that incarcerated women, who have lower incomes than incarcerated men, have an even harder time affording money bail. When the typical bail amounts to a full year's income for women, it's no wonder that women are stuck in jail awaiting trial.
>
> *(Kajstura, 2019)*

Reporting on the high number of incarcerated girls in the USA Kajstura (2019) pointed out that 10 per cent of girls are in youth facilities, were held for 'running away, truancy, and incorrigibility' (compared to boys at less than 3 per cent). It was noted that such offenses often relate to experiences of abuse and that girls of colour and LGBTQ-identified girls are disproportionately confined. They further reported that although 'LBTQ women are also disproportionately represented in the adult correctional systems', 40 per cent of girls 'in the juvenile justice system are lesbian, bisexual, or questioning and gender non-conforming' (compared to boys at just under 14 per cent) (Kajstura, 2019). As the USA has the highest incarceration rate in the world (more than one-third of the global number of incarcerated women) these insights represent deep problems of gender inequality, feminised poverty, and failures in social welfare. This extends well beyond incarceration as around two million women and girls are released from incarceration each year in the USA, meaning three out of four women under the control of any

U.S. correctional system are on probation (Kajstura, 2019). Often presented as an alternative to incarceration, women on probation face demanding conditions to avoid incarceration, including costly fees, and childcare and transportation costs for meetings with probation officers. Further, limited post-release programs are available to women due to most having been incarcerated in local jails rather than large prisons that have better facilities and funding for post-release programmes; consequently, they face a high likelihood of homelessness (Kajstura, 2019).

Although focused on the USA, many of the issues raised in that context would apply across the world and provide important insights into criminal justice for feminist practice in social welfare as it points to the structural impediments to equal justice and the need for practice and policies that aim to negotiate the complex historical and contemporary barriers to equal justice for women. The adverse conditions that women face in the prison system worldwide prompted the United Nations to create 'Rules for the Treatment of Women Prisoners and Non-custodial Measures for Women Offenders', known and applied as the Bangkok Rules (UNODC, 2011; Penal Reform International, 2013). Penal Reform International (2021) pointed out that a large proportion of women in prison are there as a 'direct or indirect result of multiple layers of discrimination and deprivation', mainly commit petty crimes related to poverty, that 'a small minority are convicted of violent offences and a large majority have been victims of violence', and that 80 per cent of women in prison have an identifiable mental illness. They also reported that in many countries women prisoners are more stigmatised than men therefore are not as frequently visited and 'are often rejected by their communities and even by their families, and struggle to rebuild their lives socially and economically' (Penal Reform International, 2021).

Women's prisons are both a site of and for feminist practice. The practices relate to specific demands to improve conditions, such as the availability of sanitary products for women prisoners and wider reformist demands such as anticarceral activism or specific accommodation for mothers in prisons. Castillo for example, engaged in a project with Indigenous and mestiza women in a Mexican prison whom she saw as 'victims of a penal state that criminalizes poverty and social protest' (2015, p. 155). Using oral histories of the incarcerated women, Castillo (2015) engaged with women to develop a destabilisation strategy to confront colonial, racist and sexist discourses within the penal system. A key observation in her feminist research was the creation of a 'sisterhood' amongst the diverse groups of women in the prison who were able to use the oral histories of coloniality to demonstrate how Indigenous peasant women had been excluded from access to justice (2015, p. 156). Through collaboration with an existing editorial group of non-Indigenous women already engaged in workshops (and through publications, had achieved justice for some women who were unjustly imprisoned), who agreed to work with Indigenous inmates in writing their histories, Castillo (2015) was able to make connections with a global network seeking to bring social justice into prisons.

Conclusion

I acknowledge that the field of concerns that this chapter has covered is limited in relation to the broad topic of women, criminal justice, and the law. It is an enormous field for women's experiences and feminist action and support at local, national, and global levels. There are important discussions untouched in this chapter. For example, the status, debates, and experiences relating to sex work, sex trafficking and criminalisation of sexuality, which no doubt deserve an entire chapter, especially as it is an area of intense debate between differing feminist perspectives. What I have tried to do, however, is account for and recognise issues that intersect with and include people who have been criminalised as sex workers and have diverse sexual identities. Another area that is a significant field of law and justice, which has been touched upon in earlier chapters, is the policing and impositions in family law and child protection. This field affects women disproportionally due to their greater likelihood of being sole parents, experiencing poverty or a history of abuse, experiencing domestic and family violence and their gendered role as a primary carer in most families across the world. The way families are policed has added complexity for many Indigenous peoples who have endured colonial rule and deliberate attempts to destroy their communities through the historical statutory theft and ongoing removal of children (AIATSIS, 2022; AIFS, 2020; Fasta and Collin-Vézina, 2019; Menzies, 2019), as well as the failures to have equal protection from the law due to racism and economic marginalisation.

Feminist practices within political and legislative processes have been crucial in winning greater equality for women, at differing levels of success, in most countries. Feminist politicians, lawyers, researchers, and activists have worked collaboratively across wide dimensions of criminal and social justice domains to achieve parity within the law and in the criminal justice system. However, what is clear, are the many sites in the global South and the global North where women and LGBTQI people endure inequalities that relate to gendered discrimination, gendered violence, and gendered poverty with established links to the level of available social welfare. The deeply entrenched patriarchal foundations of the judiciary, laws, policing and punishments are monumental challenges that feminists have had to, and continues to confront as service providers, advocates and professionals. The success in improving gender equality in the law and criminal justice relies very much on the participation of women in formal politics, government, policymaking, advocacy and practice, including political confrontation and breaking laws to achieve better laws.

Although the lack of justice varies across local and national communities, there is ample evidence that sexist decisions and behaviours are often mediated by the powerful privilege of 'founding fathers', colonial rulers, and everyday patriarchs. The broad feminist ambitions against sexism have motivated activism to disrupt given hierarchies of male privilege from within family and personal relations, in traditional practices, in criminal justice, the law, and policing. As discussed in this chapter, human rights and social justice frame many of these struggles with the aim of achieving bodily, social and economic autonomy for people excluded from such due to unequal gendered experiences. Addressing sex discrimination, ensuring safe, legal access to abortion, addressing justice in crimes of sexual assault and domestic violence, and changing gendered differences in incarceration are key issues discussed in this chapter and demonstrate how and where feminist praxis can be applied in the law and the criminal justice system. In intimate and public ways, these are areas of grave importance in social welfare.

Note

1 Russell (2019) reported that 'despite the steady erosion of abortion rights in conservative Republican states, national support for the *Roe v Wade* ruling is strong'. Citing NBC/*Wall Street Journal* poll from 2018, 71 per cent of Americans (including 52 per cent of Republicans) – 'didn't believe *Roe v Wade* should be overturned: the highest level of support since that poll began in 2005'. In Australia, a medical study reported that 87 per cent indicated that abortion should be lawful in at least some circumstances in the first trimester (de Crespigny et al., 2010).

References

AIATSIS (The Australian Institute of Aboriginal and Torres Strait Islander Studies) (2022) *The Stolen Generations*. Canberra: The Australian Government. https://aiatsis.gov.au/explore/stolen-generations.

AIFS (Australian Institute of Family Studies) (2020) *Child Protection and Aboriginal and Torres Strait Islander Children*. Canberra: Australian Government. https://aifs.gov.au/cfca/publications/child-protection-and-aboriginal-and-torres-strait-islander-children.

Albertyn, C. (2011) Law, gender and inequality in South Africa. *Oxford Development Studies*, 39 (2), 139–162.

Aspinwall, N. (2019) Manila's abortion ban is killing women. *Foreign Policy Magazine*, May 29. https://foreignpolicy.com/2019/05/29/manilas-abortion-ban-is-killing-women/.

Atkins, S. and Hoggett, B. (1984) *Women and the Law*. London: Basil Blackwell Ltd.

AVAAZ (2022) End the Ban against Women. AVAAZ Petition Website. https://secure.avaaz.org/campaign/en/honduras_women_loc/?bSfKqib&v=138440&cl=19148519574&_checksum=70e93bcbfd7504da42de71cc2ca0e7caea49c42531128f23fed5a2aadf67dec.

Bellinger, N. (2018) India has a sexual assault problem that only women can fix. *The Conversation*, August 27. http://theconversation.com/india-has-a-sexual-assault-problem-that-only-women-can-fix-101366.

Bernadi, B., Boughter, D., Brown, S., Dunham, A., Galietta, E., Keiper, L. and Montero, D. (2012) Abortion, partial-birth abortion, and adolescent access to abortion: An overview for social workers. *Journal of Human Behavior in the Social Environment*, 22 (8), 947–959.

Bingenheimer, J. and Skuster, P. (2017) The foreseeable harms of Trump's global gag rule. *Studies in Family Planning*, 48 (3), 279–290.

Brice, M. and Wroughton, L. (2019) U.S. expands abortion 'gag rule,' cuts funding to regional bloc: Pompeo. *Reuters*, March 27. https://www.reuters.com/article/

us-usa-abortion-pompeo/us-expands-abortion-gag-rule-cuts-funding-to-regional-bloc-pompeo-idUSKCN1R71LZ.

Bronitt, S. and Misra, A. (2014) Reforming sexual offences in India: Lessons in human rights and comparative law. *Griffith Asia Quarterly*, 2 (1), 37–56.

Castillo, R.A.H. (2015) Social justice and feminist activism: Writing as an instrument of collective reflection in prison spaces. *Social Justice*, 42 (3–4), 155–169.

Center for Reproductive Rights (2015) *Targeted Regulation of Abortion Providers (TRAP).* New York: Center for Reproductive Rights, August 28. https://www.reproductiverights.org/project/targeted-regulation-of-abortion-providers-trap.

Center for Reproductive Rights (2021) *Biden Administration Rescinds Global Gag Rule.* New York: Center for Reproductive Rights. https://reproductiverights.org/biden-administration-rescinds-global-gag-rule/.

Cooper, C. (2022) Women judges mobilize to help endangered Afghan counterparts. *American Bar Association.* https://www.americanbar.org/groups/diversity/women/publications/perspectives/2022/february/women-judges-mobilize-help-endangered-afghan-counterparts/.

Cormack, L. (2021) Landmark sexual consent laws pass NSW Parliament. *The Sydney Morning Herald*, November 23. https://www.smh.com.au/politics/nsw/massively-satisfied-landmark-sexual-consent-laws-pass-nsw-parliament-20211123-p59bho.html.

de Crespigny, L.J., Wilkinson, D.J., Douglas, T., Textor, M. and Savulescu, J. (2010) Australian attitudes to early and late abortion. *Australian Medical Journal*, 193 (1), 9–12.

Fasta, E. and Collin-Vézina, D. (2019) Historical trauma, race-based trauma, and resilience of indigenous peoples: A literature review. *First Peoples Child and Family Review*, 14 (1), 166–182.

Frayer, L. (2022) Marital rape is still legal in India. A court decision could change that. NPR (National Public Radio) Goats and Soda Report, USA. https://www.npr.org/sections/goatsandsoda/2022/02/08/1047588035/marital-rape-india.

Gabrielson, A. and Milender, P. (2013) Abortion. *Georgetown Journal of Gender and the Law*, 14 (2), 213–243.

Global Fund for Women (2022) *How the "Green Wave" Movement Achieved a Historic Win for Abortion Rights in Mexico.* San Francisco, CA: Global Fund for Women. https://www.globalfundforwomen.org/latest/article/how-the-green-wave-movement-achieved-an-historic-win-for-abortion-rights-in-mexico/.

Greer, G. (2018) *Germaine Greer on Rape.* London: Bloomsbury Publishing.

Gross, K.N. (2015) African American women, mass incarceration, and the politics of protection. *Journal of American History*, 102 (1), 25–33.

Heimer, K., Johnson, K., Lang, J., Rengifo, A. and Stemen, D. (2012) Race and women's imprisonment: Poverty, African American presence and social welfare. *Journal of Quantitative Criminology*, 28, 219–244.

Hungarian Spectrum (2017) The Hungarian government chips away at the abortion law. *The Hungarian Spectrum, Reflections on Politics, Economic and Culture.* https://hungarianspectrum.org/2017/02/10/the-hungarian-goverment-chips-away-at-the-abortion-law/

Jeffries, S. (2014) The imprisonment of women in Southeast Asia: Trends, patterns, comparisons and the need for further research. *Asian Journal of Criminology*, 9 (4), 253–269.

Jeffries, S. and Newbold, G. (2015) Analysing trends in the imprisonment of women in Australia and New Zealand. *Psychiatry, Psychology and Law*, 23 (2), 184–206.

Karp, P. (2019) Scott Morrison wants women to rise but not solely at expense of others. *The Guardian*, March 8. https://www.theguardian.com/world/2019/mar/08/scott-morrison-wants-women-to-rise-but-not-solely-at-expense-of-others.

Kajstura, A. (2019) Women's mass incarceration: The whole pie 2019. *Reports*. Prison Policy Initiative. https://www.prisonpolicy.org/reports/pie2019women.html.

Kennedy, P. (2020) The rape kit's secret history. *The New York Times*, June 17. (Accessed June 22, 2020). https://www.nytimes.com/interactive/2020/06/17/opinion/rape-kit-history.html.

Lang, A. (2022) First day of affirmative consent laws in NSW. *The Australian*, June 1. https://www.theaustralian.com.au/breaking-news/first-day-of-affirmative-consent-laws-in-nsw/news-story/f431e4197e7fb12fe5eaeaa41cb69d9d.

Menzies, K. (2019) Forcible separation and assimilation as trauma: The historical and socio-political experiences of Australian Aboriginal people. *Social Work & Society*, 17 (1), 1–18 (Online). https://ejournals.bib.uni-wuppertal.de/index.php/sws/index.

Ministry of Health and Family Welfare (2021) *National Family Health Survey, 2019–2021*. Mumbai: Ministry of Health and Family Welfare. http://rchiips.org/nfhs/factsheet_NFHS-5.shtml.

Olivio, A. (2021) Judges from around the world work to save female Afghan colleagues amid waning hope. *The Washington Post*, August 28. https://www.washingtonpost.com/local/afghan-women-judges-rescue/2021/08/28/ccd94798-075c-11ec-a654-900a78538242_story.

Penal Reform International (2013) UN Bangkok rules on women offenders and prisoners, short guide. https://www.penalreform.org/resource/united-nations-bangkok-rules-women-offenders-prisoners-short/.

Penal Reform International (2021) Women, key facts. https://www.penalreform.org/issues/women/key-facts/.

Rashid, R. (2022) 'Devastated': Gender equality hopes on hold as 'anti-feminist' voted South Korea's president. *The Guardian* (Online March 11, 2022). https://www.theguardian.com/world/2022/mar/11/south-korea-gender-equality-anti-feminist-president-yoon-suk-yeol.

Ratelle, N. (2018) A positive right to abortion: rethinking Roe v. Wade in the context of medication abortion. *Georgetown Journal of Gender and the Law*, 20 (1), 195–214.

Reagan, L.J. (1997) *When Abortion Was a Crime: Women, Medicine, and Law in the United States, 1867–1973*. Berkeley: University of California Press.

Russell, L. (2019) Trump (and Pence) versus women's health. *Inside Story*. Melbourne: Swinburne University. https://insidestory.org.au/trump-and-pence-versus-womens-health/.

SARA (2019) *Sexual Assault Report Anonymously*. South-Eastern Centre against Sexual Assault. https://www.sara.org.au/.

Sawer, M. (2016) The long, slow demise of the "marriage bar". *Inside Story*. Swinburne University of Technology, December 8. https://insidestory.org.au/the-long-slow-demise-of-the-marriage-bar/.

Shin, H. (2022) South Korea president-elect's pledge to shutter gender ministry stirs debate. *Reuters* (Online March 19, 2022). https://www.reuters.com/world/asia-pacific/skorea-president-elects-pledge-shutter-gender-ministry-stirs-debate-2022-03-18/.

Sommer, U. and Forman-Rabinovici, A. (2019). *Producing Reproductive Rights: Determining Abortion Policy Worldwide*. Cambridge: Cambridge University Press.

Starrs, A.M. (2017) The Trump global gag rule: an attack on US family planning and global health aid. *The Lancet*, February 4. https://www.thelancet.com/journals/lancet/article/PIIS0140-6736(17)30270-2/fulltext.

Temkin, J. (2002) *Rape and the Legal Process*. Oxford; New York: Oxford University Press.

Ting, I., Scott, N. and Palmer, A. (2020) Rough justice: How police are failing survivors of sexual assault. *ABC News, Digital Story Innovation Team* (Updated February 3, 2020). (Accessed June 22, 2020). https://www.abc.net.au/news/2020-01-28/how-police-are-failing-survivors-of-sexual-assault/11871364?nw=0.

Tippett, E. (2018) The legal implications of the MeToo movement. *Minnesota Law Review*, 103 (1), 229–302.

UNODC (United Nations Office of Drugs and Crime) (2011) The Bangkok Rules: United Nations Rules for the Treatment of Women Prisoners and Non-custodial Measures for Women Offenders with Their Commentary. United Nations General Assembly, Sixty-fifth Session. https://www.unodc.org/documents/justice-and-prison-reform/Bangkok_Rules_ENG_22032015.pdf.

United Nations (2014) *Abortion Policies and Reproductive Health Around the World*. New York: United Nations Department of Economics and Social Affairs. https://www.un.org/en/development/desa/population/publications/pdf/policy/AbortionPolcies ReproductiveHealth.pdf

United Nations (2007) Violence against women in Korea and its indicators. *Working Paper 10*. Expert Group Meeting on Indicators to Measure Violence against Women, United Nations Statistical Commission and Economic Commission for Europe and The United Nations Division for the Advancement for Women. https://www.un.org/womenwatch/daw/egm/vaw_indicators_2007/papers/Invited%20Paper%20Korea%20Whasoon%20Byun,.pdf.

UN Women (2016) *Progress of the World's Women 2015–2016, Summary*. New York: UN Women. www.unwomen.org/en/digital-library/publications/2015/4/progress-of-the-worlds-women-2015#view.

Valenti, J. (2019) Anti-abortion lawmakers have no idea how women's bodies work. *Gen*. https://gen.medium.com/anti-abortion-lawmakers-have-no-idea-how-womens-bodies-work-3ebea9fd6015.

Walker, S. (2018) Hungary passes 'slave law' prompting fury among opposition MPs. *The Guardian*, December 13. https://www.theguardian.com/world/2018/dec/12/hungary-passes-slave-law-prompting-fury-among-opposition-mps.

Webster, K., Honey, N. Mannix, S., Mickle, J, Morgan, L. Parkes, A., Politoff, V., Powell, A., Stubbs, J. and Ward, A. (2018) *Australian's Attitudes to Violence against Women and Gender Equality, Findings from the 2017 National Community Attitudes towards Violence against Women Survey*. Research Report. Sydney: ANROWS (Australia's National Research Organisation for Women's Safety).

Weil, S. and Mitra vom Berg, N. (2016) Femicide of girls in contemporary India. *ex æquo*, 34, 31–43.

Wilson, M., Simpson, P., Butler, t., Richter, J, Yap, L. and Donavan, B. (2017) 'You're a woman, a convenience, a cat, a poof, a thing, an idiot': Transgender women negotiating sexual experiences in men's prisons in Australia. *Sexualities*, 20 (3), 380–402.

Wolitzky-Taylor, K.B., Resnick, H.S., McCauley, J.L., Amstadter, A.B., Kilpatrick, D.G. and Ruggiero K.J. (2011) Is reporting of rape on the rise? A comparison of women with reported versus unreported rape experiences in the national women's study-replication. *Journal of Interpersonal Violence*, 26 (4), 807–832.

Wrack (2021) Female athletes from Afghanistan leave Kabul after being granted Australian visas. *The Guardian*, August 24. https://www.theguardian.com/world/2021/aug/24/female-athletes-from-afghanistan-leave-kabul-airport-after-being-granted-australian-visas.

World Bank (2019) *Women, Business and the Law 2019, A Decade of Reform*. Washington, DC: International Bank for Reconstruction and Development, The World Bank. https://openknowledge.worldbank.org/bitstream/handle/10986/31327/WBL2019.pdf.

8

CONCLUSION

The Fourth Wave and Feminist Practice

Introduction

In focusing on feminist practice as a form of praxis, the core project of this book has been to make connections between feminism as a social justice approach and the activities and achievements of feminists across a range of core social welfare domains. The inclusion of global South and global North perspectives provides a global point of view and, despite this being a white feminist book, to recognise and build knowledge from global South feminist praxis and, hopefully, disrupt white feminist hegemony in this field. Previous chapters have captured two important characteristics of feminism when considered as a collection of diverse and subtly different lenses for seeing the world as well as informing action towards changing the world. Therefore, as much as I have written about a singular, broad feminist commitment, an important understanding is that there are many diverse feminisms. Feminisms can be specified and distinguished by their theoretical, cultural, geographical and political underpinnings but when it comes to practice there is a broad uniformity in purpose, the challenge to end sexism and gendered oppressions and establish gender equality.

As noted earlier, using the concept of waves of feminism is not an adherence to separate phases or dissected chronologies of feminist practice and action but rather a means of establishing a broad capture of feminisms' unique developments, overlapping commitments and lively transformations in chronological contexts. In the context of this book and my experiences of feminism as both theory and practice, the fourth wave is relative to the post-1990s, a period when the third wave and its attendant postmodern turn were applied and celebrated as the framework for changes in feminist theory and practice, and the new millennium. What has emerged following the third wave is beginning to be recognised

DOI: 10.4324/9781315625188-8

as a new, fourth wave with distinct drivers and motivations based on significant transformations that have occurred in wider social, political and legal contexts, many of them related to the successes of feminist demands and actions. This chapter is dedicated to capturing, to some extent, how the fourth wave is being expressed, applied and understood.

The Fourth Wave

If pushed to define what the fourth wave looks like, I would say that it encompasses the praxis of what younger feminists are doing and theorising now, located and articulated broadly in the second and third decades of the 21st century. The single most obvious, practical characteristic of fourth-wave feminist praxis, as with other contemporary social movements, is the influence and application of communications technologies and the advent and proliferation of social media. The capacity for rapid organisation and wide collaboration has opened new opportunities for solidarity and access to shared ideas and action as well as informing us of who in the world is excluded from the benefits of our actions and ideas. In a 'big data' study that collected over one million Tweets and re-Tweets (messages on the social media platform Twitter), research showed the strength of the fourth wave as a democratising process for specific issues (Gnedash, 2022). This was explained as a process in which the Internet-based fourth wave was able to convert feminist political capital from online to offline activities, citing, for example, the #Metoo protests, global support for the rights of the women of Afghanistan in the aftermath of the Taliban overthrow of the government in 2021 and the abortion law reforms in Texas in 2021 (Gnedash, 2022).

However, along with the online strategic advances in feminist practice, has come the predictable backlash, expressed through a litany of men's anti-feminism and misogyny. This sphere of men's action against feminists and women more generally is thoroughly illuminated by Debbie Ging and Eugenia Siapera in their book, *Gender Hate Online, Understanding the New Anti-feminism*. They observe of its nature that:

> While pre-internet anti-feminism tended to mobilize men around issues such as divorce, child custody and the feminization of education, using conventional political methods such as public demonstrations and petitions, the new anti-feminists have adopted a highly personalized style of politics that often fails to distinguish between feminists and women. This is largely due to their espousal of certain essentialist and universalizing beliefs, for example, that all women are biologically destined to seek out alpha males but will exploit beta males for money, and—paradoxically— that most Western women, often referred to as "Ameriskanks", have been infected by feminism and must either be subdued or abandoned.
>
> *(2019, p. 3)*

Backlashes against feminism have always been there, but in the online environment, the violent, murderous and deeply offensive attacks demonstrate how threatened men are by the power women use and exercise for an unconstrained audience via social media and the capacity to dispense analysis and information to a global audience. Including authors from around the world, Ging and Siapera's edited book (2019) demonstrates what they see as efforts by men to 'cumulatively and forcefully violently subordinate women and seek to hinder their struggles for emancipation' (2019, p. 10). Much of the abuse has the same impact as direct forms of domestic violence, it is not just words. One chapter in their book documents, however, feminist practice that effectively uses technologies to address gendered violence through publicised lists of offenders and creating 'GIFs' (memes or symbols) that effectively express the anger felt by feminists in the online environment (Ging and Siapera, 2019, p. 11). Ging and Siapera raise some important questions for fourth-wave activists about appropriate tactics for online activism and whether this is enough. They suggest that, overall, feminism is at a critical phase and that there might be a need for 'a renewal for feminist theory and praxis', suggesting that such a development might need to begin from the bottom up (Ging and Siapera, 2019). This position reflects the nature of feminist praxis, pushing forward to open new dimensions for practice and social justice.

From a positive perspective, the technology-driven characteristic of the fourth wave is particularly evident in the statistics and analyses of women's social welfare experiences and needs, which, in this era of global action, are highly visible and valuable tools for policy change and feminist activism. Alongside this practical characteristic are the predominant lenses that feminist ideas bring to a fourth wave. Amongst scholars and within the voices and actions of younger activists, intersectionality is seen to be central to contemporary feminist perspectives, in addition to the inclusivity of gender diversity or what can be seen as the fluidity of the notion of gender and sexuality as well as body, period and gender positivity. Despite a view of globalised popular feminism as captured by and aligned with neoliberalism (Phipps, 2020), is there a capacity to share ideas and build solidarity as a movement outside neoliberal (as or and white feminist) dominance? What is new and difficult to measure is how the brevity of some feminist social media effectively educates younger women and girls to adopt feminist practice, rather than simply identify as feminist because celebrities do. For example, TikTok and Instagram host feminist 'influencers' (such as populist icons like Kim Kardashian) and more politically oriented activists such as Tilly Lawless, a Sydney-based sex worker and writer, who uses Instagram to promote feminist perspectives to her 50,000 followers, which she identifies as fourth-wave feminism (Maley, 2021). Lawless claimed that fourth-wave feminism is not just about supporting people because of their gender and that despite the extreme brevity of posts, which she states need to have some nudity to attract interest, educates young people, hopefully leading them to build more feminist knowledge (Maley,

2021). UN Women have also promoted feminist activists utilising social media as a form of activism, for example in writing about Dina Samilove who opened a dialogue about rape in Kazakhstan:

> In 2016, Smailova broke her silence by telling her story in a Facebook post. Women immediately began commenting and sending her private messages about their own experiences with violence. The outpouring of stories from others made Dina realize how important it was to keep the conversation going.
>
> "For the first time in Kazakhstan, we started talking openly about the issue, at the highest levels of the government and in the remote villages and towns, where we organized public awareness events," Smailova said. "Our movement helped other survivors of sexual abuse break their silence, report the abuse and win their cases."
>
> Now, as one of the leading figures in ending sexual violence in Kazakhstan, Dina has supported and guided more than 200 women survivors of violence and has been instrumental in winning sexual violence court cases.
>
> "I want to help more women speak out and change the attitudes within our communities. We are not the ones to be shamed! Our attackers should be ashamed and prosecuted," she said.
>
> *(UN Women, 2018)*

Like many determining analyses, both intersectionality and gender inclusivity have emerged as critical discourses and actions, and demonstrate fissures or failures in feminisms, particularly those widely circulated by hegemonic white feminist praxis. This has been demonstrated repeatedly in relation to a broad social movement action and highly politicised debates greedily circulated by dominant conservative media and extensive social media platforms. For example, despite the global reach and apparently unifying 'Pink Pussy Hats' protests (2017 & 2018) against President Trump's misogyny, criticism emerged about the dominance of white middle-class feminists in the organisation, promotion and leadership in those protests, particularly in the USA. From within, the predominance of white middle-class women's leadership and participation and the widely adopted Pink Pussy Hats that became the emblem of the protests, were seen as a failure of understanding 'intersectionalism' and gender diversity. One criticism about why this event automatically excluded women of colour was based on the colour pink, as pink relates to white skin and was seen as excluding women of colour (Compton, 2018).

Further exclusion was reported and explained in detail in the online magazine 'Seventeen' that has a very wide readership of over 4 million young people, which, according to a marketing expert (Gaille, 2015) includes a large proportion of Hispanic and teenage black subscribers. In an article entitled *'Please Stop Wearing Those Pussy Hats to Women's Marches'*, transgender-identified Mandler wrote 'when it comes down to it, not all women have vaginas and not all people with vaginas are women' (2019). The social media response and dominant media reporting highlighted the nature of fourth-wave feminism, whilst pushback against criticism of the pink hats stated that the colour pink was a reclaiming of the gendered femininity attached to the colour pink. Compton (2018) also reported about a 24-year-old protester in New York who held a sign that stated, 'Support Your Sisters, not just your Cis-ters', an implied criticism of cisgendered people excluding transgender people. Highlighting again the need for a more contemporary (fourth wave?) view she went on to say; 'I made this sign because if you're a feminist and your feminism is not intersectional, it's not feminism'. This comment caused me to reflect on my early feminist activist days when I often encountered separatist feminist claim, with which I was an alongside activist, that if you were not a lesbian then you could not be a feminist. Even though I did not identify as a lesbian, but was most certainly a feminist, I understood it was based on a well-argued view of sexism, misogyny and violence against women as perpetuated by men. Therefore, from that perspective, if you were intimate with men then you were a collaborator and part of the problem. What is important to acknowledge is that extreme views, views that create exclusions, are important in any social movement as they create dimensions for debate, action and practice and force a flexibility into debates about who is excluded when the boundaries of collective action are limited by a very specific identity.

Intersectionality

Before the specific term intersectionality became a contemporary feminist imperative, the idea of an intersection of factors, identities or conditions had long been a part of many feminist approaches and analyses. For example, Englishwoman Harriet Martineau, an early feminist sociologist (also regarded as possibly the first sociologist) had, in her early research, examined promises of equality in USA society and researched socio-political and religious social development (Arni and Müller, 2004). In one study (1838–1839), which set out to reveal conditions for women servants, she recognised the 'ubiquity of unequal social relations' such as class, sex and race (Arni and Müller, 2004). Intersectionality has become a broadly applicable term across feminist and broader social justice discourses and practices, achieving a central place in fourth-wave feminism. This is attributable to the transformation in feminism brought about by black, postcolonial and diverse women's critical voices as it also gave a name to the failures of white-dominated feminism to recognise difference in lived experiences that have overlapping causes for marginalisation, such as race, gender, sexuality, age, poverty, ableism, lack of access to education and so on. Kimberlé Crenshaw (1991), as the originator of the term, established its conceptualisation as very specific to her activism and scholarship about black women and domestic violence in the USA. However, she also sees it as 'one of many registers through which women of color boldly speak back against their theoretical marginality' (Crenshaw, 2010, p. 152). When asked what intersectionality meant to her in 2020, she stated:

> It's not identity politics on steroids...It's basically a lens, a prism, for seeing the way in which various forms of inequality often operate together and exacerbate each other. We tend to talk about race inequality as separate from inequality based on gender, class, sexuality, or immigrant status. What's often missing is how some people are subject to all of these, and the experience is not just the sum of its parts.
>
> *(Steinmetz, 2020)*

Crenshaw continued to make it clear that intersectionality is not a new form of feminism or feminist praxis, as she reasserts the fundamental social justice objectives of feminism as recognising the gendered nature of US society that, for example, sees citizenship as defined by what men and boys experience, pay inequality for women and the feminisation of poverty (Steinmetz, 2020). In other words, the fourth wave may see it as a form of feminist identity but for Crenshaw, it is a lens that provides inclusivity in feminist practice, the practice of fighting against sexism and racism in the law, in policy, welfare services and in everyday life. It is this lens of intersectionality that I have tried to incorporate throughout this book, where even though the focus may be on the long-held concerns affecting women generally, it is never a one-size-fits-all picture, and as with all social issues, context, privilege, advantage and access to resources or services are demonstrably complicated by the intersection of several disadvantages or identities.

Despite this commentary on Crenshaw's intended meanings for intersectionality, I acknowledge that it has been adopted as an imperative of contemporary or new generational, fourth-wave feminist identity. I too have embraced the logic of this important lens, which is a core part of how we understand and examine contemporary social welfare, particularly in relation to its analysis and theorisation, and need and practice. After all, social work, my teaching discipline, has distinguished itself from other human service practices based on its view of people's lives being complex in their multiple relationships (intimate, family, community and society), and recognises that individuals are rarely only affected by a single issue or social policy problem.

Gender Inclusivity

The inclusivity of the fourth-wave feminist approach to understanding gender equality as related to all genders is also critical, particularly given the debates about transgender women. This is a confrontation for some feminists who recognise women's struggles as specifically different from non-cisgender women. Fourth wavers, if I may invoke such an identity, clearly identify the exclusion of transgender women and men with wombs from the embrace of the feminist project as one of the failures of earlier feminisms. It is and must be understood as an issue of rights and for transgender people who can face extreme oppression and violence because of their gender identity, their social exclusion and victimisation as well as extreme moral judgement by the wider heteronormative community, especially the conservative religious establishment. This has become a particularly powerful social welfare issue, as in many countries, social and legal gains have been made. This included, for example allowing transgender people to change their birth certificates (without having had surgical interventions) and to marry (Hines, 2020) and a broader shift toward recognising that children know their gender identity early in life and are being increasingly recognised as having rights to be who they know they are. Moral panic created about children being able to express their identity has been bound up with conspiracies about undue LGTBQI influence and 'corruption' has prompted conservative groups to attempt to and successfully impose legal and religious constraints on transgender women in sport (in particular), due to their 'superior strength'. This has become a flagship target of conservative attacks on transgender women that have been widely circulated. For example, Australian Prime Minister Morrison in 2022 backed a parliamentary member's Bill to 'save women's sport' by excluding transgender people from single-sex sports (Martin, 2022). Further, by 2021 this had been demonstrated through the creation and approval of laws (and many proposed laws across the USA) in ten states in the USA that exclude transgender girls from competing in women's and girls' sports (Sharrow, 2021). Elizabeth Sharrow explained:

> Republican lawmakers now aim to reframe sex non-discrimination policies as means of gendered exclusion. Such transexclusionary ideas and political agendas are not new ... but the content of current proposals reveal the centrality of the physical body itself—and body politics more generally—in shaping the future of American gender politics. Recent legislative proposals advance what I call "cisgender supremacy", a logic that inheres in political assertions about normatively gendered bodies. Political institutions have emerged as another site for advancing, enshrining, and normalizing cis–supremacist gender orders, explicitly joining cause with medical authorities as arbiters of gender normativity.
>
> *(2021, p. 2)*

It is also a focus in schools at a curriculum level and in relation to welfare for students, where books have been banned and attempts made to allow religious schools to exercise freedom to exclude LGBTQI-identified students and teaching staff. As Sharrow (2021) notes above such reactions are consistent with the hegemonic power of heteronormative expectations of how people should choose to express their gender identity as part of the anti-woke reaction to be free of a binary conceptualisation of personhood. Fourth-wave feminism identifies support for transgender, non-binary, and queer rights as a central tenet of inclusivity.

The most publicised contemporary debate within feminism, where perhaps a feminist narrative of growing up as a girl and becoming a woman has been framed by exclusive experiences and views on biological as well as social impositions, can be viewed simply from a social justice perspective, where feminism's key cause is to oppose all sexism and sexist oppression. As Zoe Williams (2020) clearly explains from a contemporary feminist point of view:

> The mainstream feminist view, which is trans-inclusive, has been sidelined to maintain the fiction that this is a generational battle between old and young feminists. Again, it is tactical and convenient to portray trans inclusion as a Trojan horse that all the young idiots allow in, being unaware of the history of women's rights. But it simply is not so. Just because you are middle aged does not mean you agree with Germaine Greer. …
>
> It is astonishing that the idea of the "women-only space" is being touted as a fundamental pillar of the movement yet is completely stripped of the historical context of that. Women-only space was a realm protected from our Harvey Weinsteins, where we could talk about our Harvey Weinsteins; it was not a hallowed place where we communicated through our ovaries. It was where we came together in unity against people who hated us. I can't imagine the mindset that would exclude a trans sister from that.

The reference to 'Harvey Weinsteins' relates to the predatory, sexually abusing men who have been outed in the '#Metoo' movement and the reference to 'safe spaces' relates to some feminists and many trans-phobic commentators objecting to transwomen using women's toilets or changerooms that are designated 'safe spaces'. Prominent feminists such as Germaine Greer who has been critical of transgender women in cisgender women's struggles and JK Rowling who supported other women with certain views about transgender women in safe spaces (Rowling, 2020), have prompted transgender women and gender-inclusive feminists to fight back against what they see as exclusion from the feminist project or the women's movement or a right to be as equal in their womanhood. This debate must not overshadow the issue of rights to be recognised and supported as a woman. Inventing the term TERF, an acronym coined by trans activists, which stands for Trans-Exclusionary Radical Feminist, and creating a blanket of criticism of some feminists, played out as a hostile political action against radical feminism and other second-wave feminists, appears to have been widely accepted by fourth wave feminists. This positioning of radical feminism is at the crux of Zoe Williams (2020) observation about creating a false generational divide between second and fourth-wave feminism. Recognition and inclusion of the rights of transgender women should enhance solidarity among feminists rather than threaten it. After all, as Sally Hines clearly argued, it was the attachment to biological differences between men and women as based on reproductive capacities in 19th century medical science that revealed diverse identities:

> Central to the formulation of sexed and gendered difference was a binary model wherein male and female were polarised. Commonalities between men and women were negated as dissimilarities were underscored. Further – and crucially – variations between the binaries of male and female became pathologised. Yet such pathologisation could not be possible without recognition of bodies – and experiences – that were beyond the binary. Thus, throughout the 19th century, bodies and identities that lay across or outside of the male/female binary became visible.
>
> *(2020, p. 701)*

For feminist practice, the welfare of transgender women is as important as the welfare of cisgender women. Although not always the case, social welfare must be all embracing, therefore services must account for the needs of specific groups and recognise the lived experience of divergent identities. After all, body positivity and sex positivity are embodied in experiential knowledge of transgender women and men (lived experiences are widely available in Ted Talks available on 'YouTube'). A shift to a visible identity as a woman, for example brings with it the experiences of heteronormative sexism in the forms of everyday harassment and feminised positioning by cisgender men. For inclusive feminist activism, transwomen's first-hand experiencing the difference between social interactions as a woman after being seen as a man in social contexts leads to observations of the impact of sexism as a distinctive experience of being a woman. This unique perspective is valuable in confronting everyday sexism.

An important consequence of widespread transphobia emerging from a deep-seated vilification of many gender non-conforming people, and a backlash against successes for transgender people gaining legal rights and public voices, are the high levels of suicide amongst transgender people and violent assaults on and murders of transgender women of colour. The USA-based NGO, Human Rights Campaign reported that in 2021, 56 transgender or gender non-conforming people were violently killed (Human Rights Campaign, 2021). This is an underestimate as often such crimes go unreported and according to their analysis, most murdered transgender people were Black and Latinx transgender women (Human Rights Campaign, 2021).

It is important for feminist practitioners to recognise the complexity of debates such as the transgender woman/cisgender conflict or divide, as social justice can only be sought if the specific oppressions that it seeks to counter are well understood. I have included the discussion above because it appears to be central to fourth-wave feminism and raises challenges for feminist solidarity and feminist practice and advocacy in social welfare. If the fourth wave seeks to be inclusive of diversity, then it faces the same challenges that hegemonic white feminism faced in previous waves. This is particularly evident when compared to core concerns of global South feminists whose struggles are predominantly focused on feminised poverty, lack of equal access to education, failures in maternal health, lack of reproductive rights, lack of representation in political and government processes, wage disparity and practices that curtail freedom. Accepting that at its core fourth wave feminism is about countering and opposing sexism, sexism against anyone who suffers it, then it must embrace the complexity of what it is like to be a woman in the entire breadth of circumstances that engage feminist practice in the global South, including the extreme exclusion and victimisation of transgender people.

Conclusion

Given my now lengthy personal and scholarly engagement with feminism, I have little need to categorise my theoretical position beyond the wide embrace of feminisms presented in this book. I have drawn together a landscape of feminist practice based on what I felt was a need to document, from an ambitiously global perspective, how feminists act and practice in support of and in relation to the broadest conceptualisation of social welfare. As I mentioned in the preface, this is a white feminist book, and does not seek to represent any specific, theoretically defined feminism, or types of feminists. What I aimed to do was to open perspectives that capture the breadth and scope of feminists' struggles, actions and strategies that counter sexist, gendered impositions in diverse contexts. I understand the diverse feminist theoretical lenses that may or may not have informed the wide-ranging examples of activism and practices I have borrowed to demonstrate how feminist practice contributes to social welfare. However, in doing so I have skirted over deeper theoretical debates about feminist theory and my own theoretical feminist anatomy and focused on the ongoing gendered social issues that continue to challenge most societies across the world. This is based on a firm belief that feminist practice always seeks social justice outcomes and seeks to contribute to building socially just communities where women and people of other genders, including men, can lead good, more equal lives, unencumbered by gendered oppressions or exclusions. This aspiration for feminist practice does align, theoretically, with a standpoint feminist position but, having been a feminist activist of radical feminism in the second wave period and engaged with the important deconstruction of universalist perspectives in the third wave period, I also align, theoretically with poststructuralist feminisms, particularly postcolonial feminism and, as noted in this chapter and through examples of practice, I also recognise and support the values and ambitions of fourth wave feminists. Although many of the chapter topics focus on the most dire or worst excesses of gender inequality and how they limit access to equal or appropriate social welfare and social justice, the key aim of this book was to demonstrate the resilience and importance of feminist practice, as praxis, and as political and cultural activism toward emancipation, in social policy change, and in welfare service delivery.

As a final observation, I would like to return to Serene Khader's (2018) critique of disjuncture between global South values related to tradition, family, community and religion with the hegemonic white liberal/neoliberal values of global North feminists, who are seen as positioning themselves as saviours of women in the global South. Khader argued in favour of a transnational feminist praxis from a global South point of view. She proposed that this reorientation would avoid re-colonising tendencies of global North feminisms, arguing that 'feminism requires universalist opposition to sexist oppression, but feminism does not require universal adoption of Western "Enlightenment liberal" values and strategies' (2018, p. 4). Given the central role neoliberalism is playing in contemporary oppressions, not just of women but inclusive of entire nations, communities and socio-economically disadvantaged individuals, this seems a position that global feminist praxis could agree upon. Khader's inherent critique of the dominance of neoliberal ideals that set out to determine 'which goods and power should be allocated' overshadows the feminist objective of ending sexist oppression, which 'mostly makes a point about how goods and power should be allocated' (2018, p. 4). Khader's (2018) analysis of the impact of uncritical assumptions about free-market capitalism benefiting women in the global South, and observations of how global North economic and social welfare interventions are imposed via the 'development' paradigm, is central to considerations for a global feminist praxis. The reorientation of perspectives in global or transnational feminism toward a global South perspective offers a way forward for the numerous historical and contemporary aspirations for a more gender-equal world. The principles of inclusivity and positivity that are at the core of contemporary (fourth-wave) feminism can be envisaged encompassing possible spaces for solidarity with global South tradition, family, community and religion. In the context of this book, this challenge seems critical if the social justice objectives of feminisms that support social welfare for all are to be met.

References

Arni, C. and Müller, C. (2004) More sociological than the sociologists? Undisciplined and undisciplinary thinking about society and modernity in the nineteenth century. In B. Marshall and A. Witz (eds) *Engendering the Social, Feminist Encounters with Sociological Theory.* New York: McGraw Hill Education, 71–92.

Compton, J. (2018) At 2nd annual Women's March, some protesters left 'pussy hats' behind. *NBCNews.*https://www.nbcnews.com/feature/nbc-out/2nd-annual-women-s-march-some-protesters-left-pussy-hats-n839901.

Crenshaw, C. (2010) Close encounters of three kinds: On teaching dominance feminism and intersectionality. *Tulsa Law Review,* 46 (1), 151–189.

Crenshaw, K. (1991) Mapping the margins: Intersectionality, identity politics, and violence against women of color. *Stanford Law Review,* 43 (6), 1241–1299.

Gaille, B. (2015) 18 great seventeen magazine demographics. *BrandonGaille Small Business and Marketing Advice.* https://brandongaille.com/18-great-seventeen-magazine-demographics/.

Ging, D. and Siapera, E. (eds) (2019) *Gender Hate Online Understanding the New Anti-Feminism*. Cham, Switzerland: Springer International Publishing, Palgrave Macmillan.

Gnedash, A.A. (2022) The fourth wave of feminism: Political discourse and opinion leaders in Twitter. *Journal of Political Science*, 24 (1), 64–89.

Hines, S. (2020) Sex wars and (trans) gender panics: Identity and body politics in contemporary UK feminism. *The Sociological Review (Keele)*, 68 (4), 699–717.

Human Rights Campaign (2021) *Fatal Violence against the Transgender and Gender Non-Conforming Community in 2021*. Human Rights Campaign. https://www.hrc.org/resources/fatal-violence-against-the-transgender-and-gender-non-conforming-community-in-2021.

Khader, S.J. (2018) *Decolonizing Universalism: A Transnational Feminist Ethic*. New York: Oxford University Press.

Maley, J. (2021) Grace Tame, TikTok and the emergence of feminism's fourth wave. *The Sydney Morning Herald*, February 20, 2022, 5.00 am. https://www.smh.com.au/politics/federal/grace-tame-tiktok-and-the-emergence-of-feminism-s-fourth-wave-20220217-p59xev.html.

Mandler, C. (2019) Please stop wearing those pussy hats to women's marches. *Seventeen*. https://www.seventeen.com/life/a15854506/stop-wearing-pussy-hats-womens-marches/.

Martin, S. (2022) Scott Morrison backs bill that allows exclusion of transgender people from single-sex sports. *The Guardian*, February 22. https://www.theguardian.com/society/2022/feb/22/scott-morrison-backs-bill-that-allows-exclusion-of-transgender-people-from-single-sex-sports.

Phipps, A. (2020) *Me, Not You: The Trouble with Mainstream Feminism*. Manchester: Manchester University Press.

Rowling, J.K. (2020) J.K. Rowling writes about her reasons for speaking out on sex and gender issues. https://www.jkrowling.com/opinions/j-k-rowling-writes-about-her-reasons-for-speaking-out-on-sex-and-gender-issues/.

Sharrow, E.A. (2021) Sports, transgender rights and the bodily politics of cisgender supremacy. *Laws*, 10 (63), 1–29.

Steinmetz, K. (2020) She coined the term 'intersectionality' over 30 years ago. Here's what it means to her today. *Time*. https://time.com/5786710/kimberle-crenshaw-intersectionality/.

UN Women (2018) Six activists who are using social media for change offline. *News and Events*, UN Women, June 29. https://www.unwomen.org/en/news/stories/2018/6/compilation-social-media-day.

Williams, Z. (2020) Feminist solidarity empowers everyone. The movement must be trans-inclusive. *The Guardian*, March 11. https://www.theguardian.com/society/2020/mar/10/feminist-solidarity-empowers-everyone-the-movement-must-be-trans-inclusive.

INDEX

ableism 6, 180
abortion: contraception and rights to
    106–113; and law 161–167
Abortion Counselling Service of the
    Chicago Women's Liberation Union 109
Abu-Lughod, Lila 52
abuse, and care 140–143
Adegoke, Yomi 103
Adoption and Safe Families Act (ASFA) 79
advocacy 10, 31; and abortion laws 165; for
    change across market 77; for feminist
    action and influence 48; for mothers 81;
    for old citizens 124; and older feminists
    144–145; political 145; radical 33; in
    social welfare 184
African American women 81–82, 85, 89
African 'womanism' 14
ageing: 'ageing in place' 138–139; 'ageing-
    well' 125; documentation of 128;
    experience for older women 131–135;
    global perspectives on 128–130;
    government policies related to 132; lived
    experiences of 124
ageism 6; critique of 146; gendered 132;
    and sexism 131–135
Albertyn, Catherine 155
al-Hathloul, Loujain 30
'alt-right' politics 6
Arab Spring 27
Arrigoitia, Melissa Fernandez 138–139
assisted reproductive technologies (ARTs)
    113–117, 119

Australian Human Rights
    Commission 126, 137
The Australian Institute of Superannuation
    Trustees 37

Baldwin, M. 145
Bangkok Rules see United Nations
    'Rules for the Treatment of Women
    Prisoners and Non-custodial
    Measures for Women Offenders'
Barry, K. 26
Baumgardner, J. 14
Bearak, J. 106
Beauvoir, Simone de 127
Beijing Platform for Action 34
Biden, Joe 165
birth parents: knowledge of
    114; transgender men as
    73–74
Blondet, Celia 144
'Bloody Good Period' 103
Boddy, J. 7
Borell, Lena 140
Bowen, S. 75
Briggs, Laura 72
British Poor Laws 11
Brooks, Kim 82–83
Browning, C.J. 125
Bryant, Phil 164
Burke, Tarana 157
Butler, Judith 14
Butler, Robert 131

Cacciatore, J. 91
Caddick, Alison 113
Calasanti, Toni 124, 132–133
Caldas-Coulthard, C. 134–135
Campoamor, Leigh 81
care and abuse 140–143
Catholicism 25, 107
Center for Disease Control and
    Prevention 82, 118
Chang, G. 12
Charpentier, M. 124, 143
Chaturvedi, S. 88
Chazan, M. 145
Chesler, Phyllis 64
childbirth 90–93
Chrisler, J. 131, 134–135
Christianity 27
Clarke, Laura Hurd 131
Collins, Judy 110
The Coming of Age (Beauvoir) 127
Connell, Raewyn 25, 32, 39
conservative politics 6
contraception and rights to abortion
    106–113
Convention on the Elimination of All
    Forms of Discrimination against Women
    (CEDAW) 50
Corea, Gena 113–115
Costello, K. 64
Covid-19 pandemic 5, 36, 48, 90, 141, 146
Cree, V.E. 9
Crenshaw, Kimberlé 180–181
criminal justice 18, 44, 47, 55, 61, 92, 151,
    153, 170

Dalvie, Suchitra 93
Daly, Mary 100
Dean, J.S. 9
de Certeau, Michel 9
De Courtivron, I. 24–25
defensive motherhood 81
'Destroy the Joint' 61–62
Dhawale, Mariam 158
Dixon, L.Z. 87
domestic violence 44–66, 151; countering
    56–60; defined 50; feminist practice
    against 46–48; and health 63–65; as
    ongoing global problem 50–56; research
    60–63; worldwide violence against
    women 48–50
Domestic Violence Prevention Act
    (Taiwan) 55
domestic violence research 60–63
Dougherty, E.N. 131
Dunkerley, S. 92
Dworkin, A. 26

economic rationalism 3
El Jaouhari, Sara 94
Elliot, S. 75
Ephron, Nora 110
Eschle, C. 23–24
Escude, M. 79
Estes, Carroll 128, 135–136
Eurocentrism 15
European Union (EU) 37
European Women's Lobby (EWL) 37
Everitt, L. 93
Eyadat, Z. 27

Faulkner, Debbie 138
Fejo-King, C. 4
feminisation of poverty 11, 36, 168, 181, 185
feminism: across the World 24–30;
    commodification of 6; fourth-wave
    14, 23, 177–180; global North 2, 40,
    186; intersectional 3; Islamic 27; liberal
    9, 32; positioning of 5–8; postcolonial
    14, 185; practicing 8–9; as praxis 1–19;
    procedural 3; radical 3; 'second wave'
    13–14; Southern 14; third-wave 14, 76;
    transnational 29; universal 29; waves of
    12–15; Western 27, 29; women and 16
'Feminist Current' 26
feminist medical doctors 93–95
feminist practice: in challenging the law
    151–153; against domestic violence
    46–48; by and for older women 143–145
feminist theory 3, 35, 94, 176, 178, 185
Firestone, Shulamith 113
'first wave' feminism 13
Fonseca, Claudia 80–81
foreign nongovernmental organisations
    (NGOs) 165
formal non-governmental organisations 31
Forman-Rabinovici, A. 167
fourth-wave feminism 14, 23, 177–180
Fourth World Conference on Women in
    Beijing (1995) 50
Fraser, Nancy 46–47

Garner, Diana 127
gender 1; alignment 16; equality 4, 22–23,
    25, 30–31, 33, 38–40, 45, 55; equality
    policies 16, 22, 36–37; identity 10, 26;
    inclusivity 18; inequality 3, 34–36, 38,
    40, 50, 56; oppression 16; roles and
    hierarchies 10; stereotypes 56
gender-based violence 50, 56, 63, 135,
    154–155
*Gender Hate Online, Understanding the
    New Anti-feminism* (Ging and
    Siapera) 177

gender inclusivity 181–185
gender power relations 56–57
gender-role elimativism 29
'gender studies' 7
Ghandi, Kirin 103
Ging, Debbie 177–178
global feminism 16, 22–40
Global Financial Crisis 37
global inequality 36–39
global neoliberalism 144
Global North 4, 10, 15, 91
global North feminisms 2, 40, 186
Global South 4, 15
global South women 2, 151
Goddard, Marty 160
Gordon, L. 11
GRAN 145
Grate, Rachel 104
Gray, M. 7
Greenwald, B.D. 64
Green Wave 166
Greer, Germaine 161, 183
Gunter, Jen 105
Gunter, Jennifer 105
Gyn/Ecology: the metaethics of radical feminism (Daly) 100–101

Haghighat, Elhum 12
health and domestic violence 63–65
HelpAge USA 133–134
Heo, MinSook 47, 57
Her 103
Herrera, Sayuri 53
Hines, Sally 183
Hodžić, S. 35
Holmstrom-Smith, A. 116, 119
homelessness 12, 17, 126, 137, 146
Honda, S. 55
honour killings 151
Honour killings 51
hooks, bell 8, 71
Hosseine, S. 90
Housing for the Aged Action Group (HAAG) 138
Htun, M. 57
Hulko, W. 8
Human Rights Campaign 184
Human Rights Watch 30

Im, Eun-Ok 105
Incarcerated Mother's Law group 79
informal non-governmental organisations 31
intensive motherhood 75
International Federation of Social Workers 101

International Monetary Fund 136
International Network of the Prevention of Elder Abuse 141
intersectional feminism 3
intersectionality 14, 180–181
Irish Women's Liberation Movement 107
Irish Women United (IWU) 106
Islam 27
Islamic feminism 27

Janani Suraksha Yojana (India) 87–88
Johansson, Karin 140
Johnson, Candace 117
Jones, Rebecca 131
Judaism 27

Kartini, Raden Adjeng 25
Kelly, Laura 107
Khader, Serene 29, 186
King, Billy Jean 110
Kuan, H. 56
Kulczycki, A. 51
Kuleshova, A. 76

The Lancet 2
law: abortion and 161–167; affecting women, changes to 153–158; feminist practices in challenging 151–153; and women 158–161
Law, V. 79
Lazar, Michelle 6
lesbian, gay, bisexual, queer, intersex and asexual (GLBTQIA+) communities 44
Lester, Laurence 138
'Letters of a Javanese Princess' (Kartini) 25
LGBTQI people 3, 170, 182
liberal feminism 9, 32
Lombardo, E. 3
Lorenz, Walter 10
Lotkeff, Lana 6

MacKinnon, C.A. 26
Maiguashca, B. 23–24
Make Mothers Matter 85
Malik, Sarah 28
Marchenko, Myroslava 113
Margaria, A. 74
Marks, E. 24–25
Martineau, Harriet 180
maternal death and abuse 81–85
maternal rights 71–95
McCormak, Jennie 162–163
McHugh, M.C. 143
McRobbie, Angela 7–8, 15
medical doctors 93–95

The Menopause Manifesto, Own Your Health with Facts and Feminism (Gunter) 105
menstruation 102–106
#MeToo movement 23, 156–158, 177, 183
Middle African Network for Women's Reproductive Health (GCG) in Gabon 111
Milano, Alyssa 157
'The Mirror of Contemplating Affairs' (Taymour) 25
Moon, R. 134–135
Morrison, Scott 154, 182
motherhood: defensive 81; impositions and expectations 74–78; intensive 75; rights 78–81
The Mother Machine: From Artificial Insemination to Artificial Wombs (Corea) 113
Moulding, N. 9
Ms. Magazine 110
Mullins, Saxon 160

National Domestic Violence Hotline (USA) 49
National Labor Relations Act Board (NLRAB) 158
Nelson, C. 75–76
neoliberalism 3, 8, 47
New French Feminisms 24
New Ground co-housing project 138–139
New South Wales Bureau of Crime Statistics and Research (NSWBCSR) 61
Niles, Mimi 89
nongovernmental organisations (NGOs) 38, 40; foreign 165; formal 31; grassroots 165; informal 31; international 165; women's/feminist 31–36

obstetric violence 85–90
O'Donnell, K.S. 109
OECD Family Data Base 126
Ogawa, R. 55
older women: feminist practice by and for 143–145; nexus of ageing experience for 131–135; and risk of poverty 135–140
Older Women's Co-housing Network (OWCH) 138–139
Ong, Aihwa 28–29
Open Line Counselling 107
Orbán, Viktor 154–155
O'Reilly, Bill 104
Our Watch 59
Oxfam 33

parents: intended 118; sole 126, 170; transgender men as birth 73–74
Patrone, Tatiana 118
Pearce, Diana 11
Penal Reform International 168
'period poverty' 103
Phillips, R. 9
Phipps, A. 23
'Pink Pussy Hats' protests 23, 179
Plan International 103
'Please Stop Wearing Those Pussy Hats to Women's Marches' (Mandler) 179
positioning of feminism 5–8
postcolonial feminism 14, 185
postfeminism 7–8, 35
poverty: feminisation of 36, 168, 181, 185; gendered risk of 38, 170; and homelessness 12, 17, 126, 146; older women and risk of 135–140; 'period poverty' 103
practicing feminism 8–9
praxis, feminism as 1–19
Prendergast, C. 110
prison system: women in 167–169
procedural feminism 3
Programme of Action of the International Conference on Population and Development 34

racism 6, 53, 75, 80, 95, 133–134, 153, 170, 181
radical feminism 3
Ratelle, Nicole 162–163
Rawlings, Linda 88
reproductive justice: assisted reproductive technologies (ARTs) 113–117, 119; contraception and rights to abortion 106–113; goal of 116–117; menstruation 102–106; policy agenda 116
'reproductive labour' 72–73
'reproductive prostitution' 118
reproductive rights 11, 13, 34, 73–74, 78, 100–101, 106–120, 165, 167
Rice, M. 55
rights: maternal 71–95; motherhood 78–81; reproductive 11, 13, 34, 73–74, 78, 100–101, 106–120, 165, 167; and welfare 100–120
rights to abortion 106–113
Robertson, R. 75–76
Roe v Wade 163
Rosche, Daniela 33
Rosenberg, Lena 140
Rowling, J.K. 183

Rudolph, Marc 104
Ruiz, A.G. 12

Samilove, Dina 179
Schurr, C. 115, 117
'second wave' feminism 13–14
Second World War 15
sexism and ageism 131–135
Sharma, Malika 94
Sharrow, Elizabeth 182
Shaw, C.M. 1
'She Decides' program 165
Siapera, Eugenia 177–178
social justice 1, 5–10, 12, 16, 22–23, 27, 35, 57, 73, 93, 95, 112, 115, 125, 143, 146
social justice activism 1
social media 5, 14, 23, 26, 28, 59, 61–62, 75, 103, 110, 132, 143, 145, 157, 161, 167–168, 177–180
social welfare 1–12, 22, 24, 34–40, 44–46, 61–62, 71–74, 95, 101, 106, 112–119, 124
Sommer, U. 167
South-Eastern Centre against Sexual Assault 161
Southern feminism 14
Stanley, Liz 2
Stern, Elizabeth 117
Stern, William 117
stranger killings 151
'stratified reproduction' 117
Suk-yeol, Yoon 154
surrogacy 117–119
Sustainable development Goals (SDGs) 165

Taliban 150, 177
Targeted Regulation of Abortion Providers (TRAP Laws) 164
Taymour, Aisha 25
Tedmanson, D. 4
Ted Talks 184
Teo, Peggy 130
third-wave feminism 14, 76
Thomson Reuters Survey 151
Tippett, E. 157–158
Trans-Exclusionary Radical Feminist 183
transgender men as birth parents 73–74
transnational feminism 29
trans parenthood 71–95
Troutman, M. 106
Trump, Donald 6, 31, 39, 72, 154, 158, 179; 'Mexico City Policy' or 'Global Gag Rule' 165; 'Pink Pussy Hats' protests 23, 179

Tulugak, Minu 83

UN Convention on CEDAW 55
United Nations (UN) 22, 140, 141; Fourth World Conference on Women in Beijing 101; Millennium Development Goals (MDGs) 32–33, 82, 87; 'Rules for the Treatment of Women Prisoners and Non-custodial Measures for Women Offenders' 169; Sustainable Development Goals (SDGs) 32–33, 38, 40, 50, 51
United Nations Office of Drugs and Crime 50
universal feminism 29
UN Women 37–38, 77, 179

Valenti, Jessica 163
Verloo, M.M. 3
violence: gender-based 50, 56, 63, 135, 154–155; obstetric 85–90
Voicu, Ilona 105
Volunteers of Legal Services 79

waves of feminism 12–15
Weldon, S.L. 57
welfare state 10, 11, 15, 36, 77, 81, 116, 119, 130, 136, 138, 140, 143
Wendt, S. 9
West, Karen 15, 138–139
Western feminisms 27, 29
Western international feminism 28
White, V. 9
Whitehead, Mary Beth 117
Wieber Lens, J. 91
Williams, Zoe 183
Windle, S. 51
womanhood, patriarchal idea of 75
women: African American 81–82, 85, 89; changes to laws affecting 153–158; with disabilities 3; and feminism 16; law fails 158–161; in prison system 167–169; worldwide violence against 48–50
women of colour 2, 3
women's/feminist NGOs 22, 23–24, 31–36
'women's liberation movement' 13
Women's Prison Association 79
World Bank 136, 156
World Economic Forum (WEF) 36, 38, 39
World Health Organisation (WHO) 22, 45, 53–54, 86, 107–109, 141, 167
'*The World's Oldest Oppression*' conference 26
worldwide violence against women 48–50

#YouKnowMe 110

For Product Safety Concerns and Information please contact our EU
representative GPSR@taylorandfrancis.com
Taylor & Francis Verlag GmbH, Kaufingerstraße 24, 80331 München, Germany

www.ingramcontent.com/pod-product-compliance
Lightning Source LLC
Chambersburg PA
CBHW070329270326
41926CB00017B/3820